THE SPIRIT OF YOGA

The Spirit of Yoga

by Cat de Rham & Michèle Gill

Thorsons

Thorsons
An Imprint of HarperCollins*Publishers*
77–85 Fulham Palace Road
Hammersmith
London W6 8JB

The Thorsons website address is:
www.thorsons.com

Published by Thorsons 2001

10 9 8 7 6 5 4 3 2 1

A catalogue record for this book is available from
the British Library

ISBN 0 00 710882 6

Printed and bound in Great Britain by
Scotprint, Haddington, East Lothian

to lightness

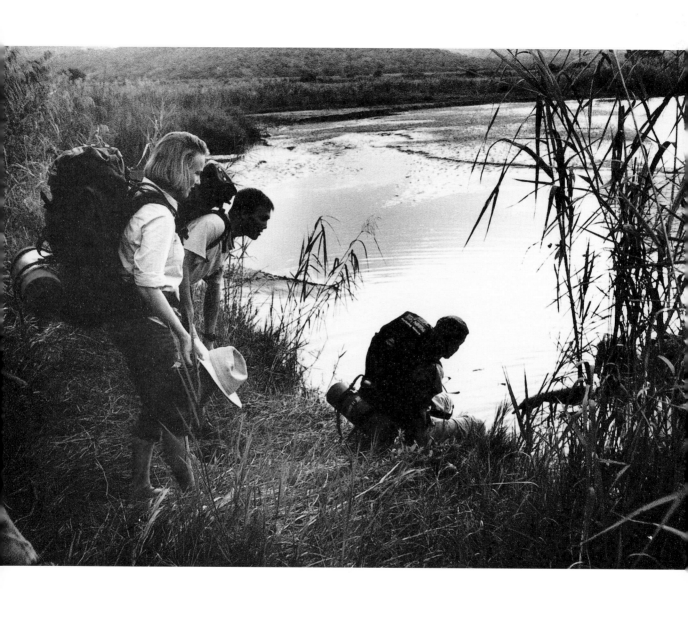

"We're all going on an Expotition with
Christopher Robin!"
"What is it when we're on it?"
"A sort of boat, I think," said Pooh.
"Oh! that sort."
"Yes. And we're going to discover a Pole
or something. Or was it a Mole?
Anyhow we're going to discover it."

A. A. MILNE

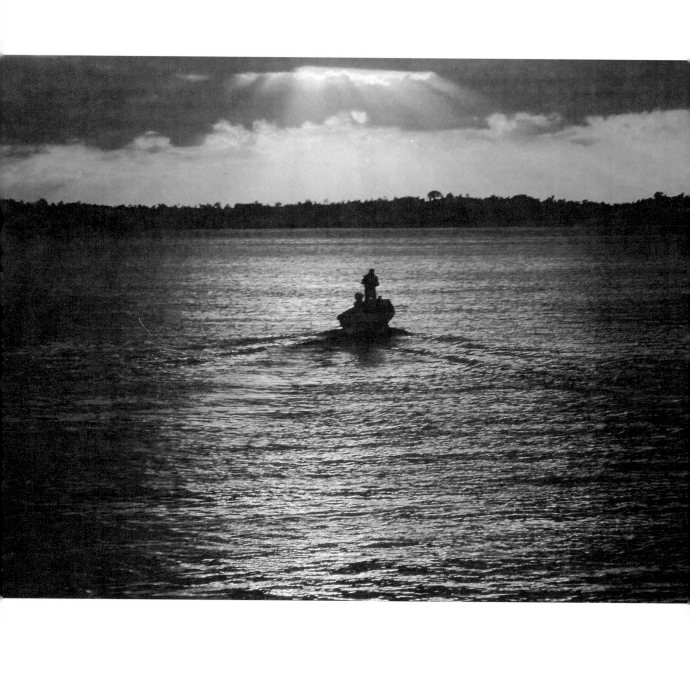

The Spirit of Yoga seeks to create a vehicle through which anyone can grasp the essence of yoga ... its meaning, relevance, and application to life today.

This is not a how-to-posture book or an abstract academic discourse. This is a book that charts the individual's discovery of yoga as a means to self-realization and a way to live your life.

We want to get across how anybody can engage in and be inspired by the old yoga texts, their wisdom, their way. How, while *samadhi* or enlightenment may only be experienced by a few, we can still all benefit immensely from the practices of yoga. They are direct. They make sense. And when practiced, they work.

You may be curious: What is yoga? With writing, poetry, and images, this book offers an accessible and illuminating exploration of the question itself.

Patanjali's Sutras

Patanjali is the father of yoga. He is thought to have lived between 500 and 200 B.C. Although we know very little about the man himself, his yoga sutras—which codify the yoga path in succinct form—are one of the most direct and powerful pathways to enlightenment.

The word sutra itself means thread. Patanjali collected a vast amount of information and threaded the essentials together with extraordinary intelligence, clarity, and compassion. Although his work has the formality of an ancient text, he is someone who has minutely studied humanity and offers us an instruction manual to the art and science of living and evolving—residing in our true essence, being our full potential—*samadhi*.

Patanjali wrote 196 sutras, which are divided into four chapters. Within this structure are eight practical steps, each one leading to the next, yet entwined and complementing each other. These are known as the eight limbs of yoga. This book directly follows Patanjali's eightfold path.

When reading through the eight limbs of Patanjali's sutras it is important to remember that each limb is but one branch of a tree.

All the different guidelines must be woven together. On their own they remain dry and academic. As a whole they reflect each other and grow together, creating a tree of overwhelming lushness and stability.

Look to experience rather than dissect each stage of the sutras. This is the true magic of yoga—being through being.

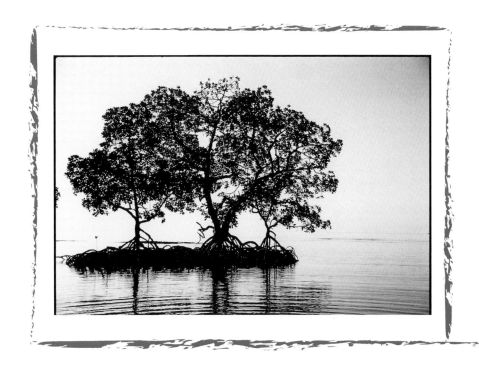

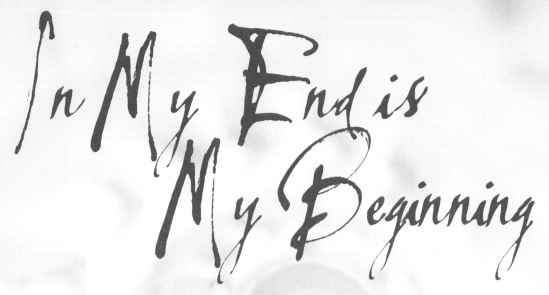

In My End is My Beginning

Yoga is the study of the infinite reality underlying the world of change. It is the path that can answer the question "Who am I?"

Throughout history people have sought to understand our core consciousness—the Self. The great sages and mystics who studied these matters found that in deep meditation, when their bodies, minds, and senses were stilled, they entered a different state. In this state they experienced a higher mode of knowing, a union with reality beyond time and change, a Self that is part of, and not separate from, this world.

The experience of this is called *samadhi*.
Living in this state continuously is called *moksha*.

Yoga is the search for this union and Patanjali's sutras are the guide to experiencing this state. Through the sutras we lead ourselves back to our source.

In our end is our beginning.

Take a Walk on the Wild Side

The eightfold path is a long and winding road that leads to a narrow and steep trail that leads to a thick and clinging forest through which you have to bushwhack in ever-increasing foreign territory before you find the clearing.

In other words, the path of yoga requires dedication, perseverance, and practice.

It helps to remember why you are practicing when the going seems tough and you are weary. Why persistence is necessary. What you are doing: Looking to meet the Giant Self.

> ... the Self is not to be found in the outside world.
> Rather it is the nucleus of our inmost being.
>
> GEORG FEUERSTEIN

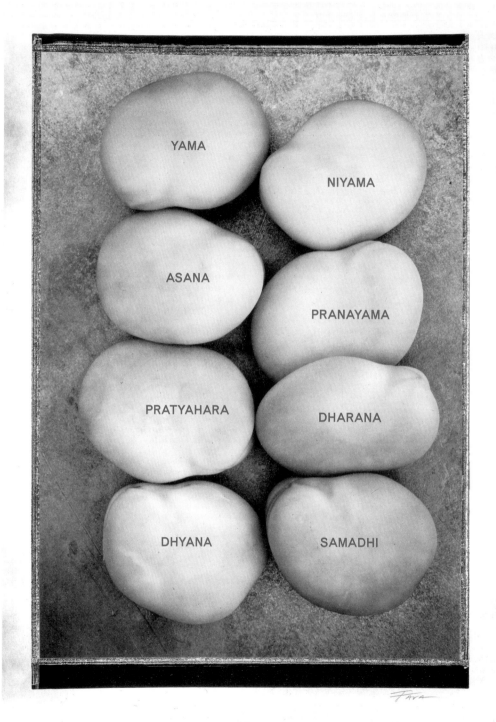

The Eight Limbs of Yoga

The eightfold path of yoga as found in Patanjali's sutras is essentially an eight-step guide to self-realization. Enlightenment.

The steps are as follows:

1. YAMA—the practice of universal moral principles

2. NIYAMA—the practice of personal disciplines

3. ASANA—the practice of physical postures

4. PRANAYAMA—the practice of breath control

5. PRATYAHARA—the practice of withdrawal of the senses

6. DHARANA—the practice of focused attention

7. DHYANA—the practice of meditation

8. SAMADHI—self-realization. Enlightenment

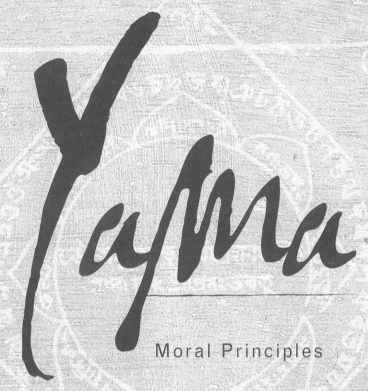

Yama

Moral Principles

Only try to know who you are. That is enough.

SRI RAMANA MAHARISHI

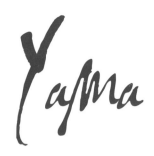

Yama is the first limb of the eightfold path of yoga. It is made up of five practices that form the ethical foundation for living one's life.

Ahimsa	Non-violence
Satya	Truth
Asteya	Non-stealing
Brahmacharya	Transforming a vital force to a spiritual level
Aparigraha	Greedlessness

The *yamas* are practices of purification. They work specifically on the mind, the seat of all our thoughts. They are in harmony with eternal and natural laws. They are guidelines for living to our greatest potential.

What is your religion telling you?
How to be a Jew? A Catholic?
Or how to be a human being?

JOSEPH CAMPBELL

2

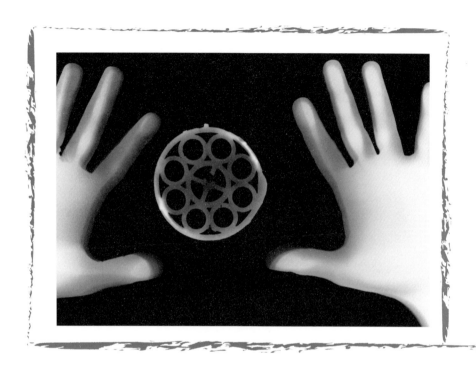

They are the ethical disciplines that show us

what must be done and what must be discarded.

They are the golden keys to unlock the spiritual gates.

B. K. S. IYENGAR

Light on the Yoga Sutras of Patanjali

Cave Meditation

Imagine a cave within yourself. A fire flickers.
On your right is Anger. Sadness to his left.
Greed sits across the circle talking to Joy and Jealousy.
Some in the group are loud and strident, blustery and strong.
Others are weaker, skinnier, with whispery voices.
It is difficult to make head or tail of what is going on.
These are your thoughts, desires, moods, judgments.

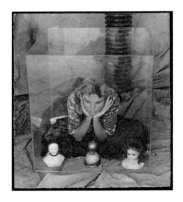

Ego, will, intellect.
This is what you think of as *you*.

But they are not you.
While your guests are parts of your mind they do not control or own you.
They need attention and understanding in equal measure.
They need acknowledgment without involvement.
Do not follow the conversation of one over the other.
Validate each one for what it is.
Learn to befriend your inner landscape with respect and compassion.
Learn to step back and be a journalist of your own mind.

The Guest House

This being human is a guest house.
Every morning a new arrival.

A joy, a depression, a meanness,
some momentary awareness comes
as an unexpected visitor.

Welcome and entertain them all!
Even if they're a crowd of sorrows,
who violently sweep your house
empty of its furniture,
still, treat each guest honorably.
He may be clearing you out
for some new delight.

The dark thought, the shame, the malice,
meet them at the door laughing,
and invite them in.

Be grateful for whoever comes,
because each has been sent
as a guide from beyond.

RUMI

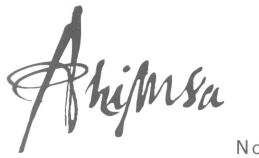

Ahimsa

Non-violence

ALL CREATION IS SACRED

Consideration for all beings.

Living in a way that causes as little harm as possible.

Cultivating love and compassion for all life.

People ask me what my religion is. I tell them, "My religion is kindness."

TENZIN GYATSO

His Holiness the XIV Dalai Lama

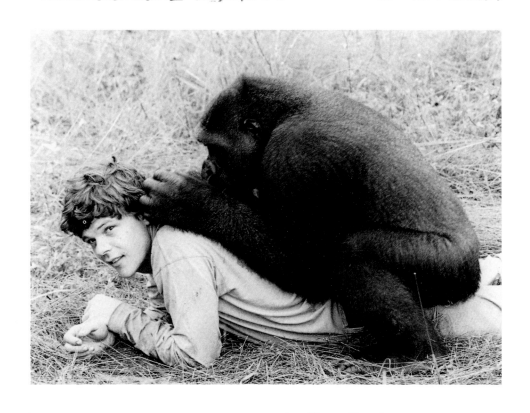

Do you know what astonished me most in the world? The inability of force to
create anything. In the long run, the sword is always beaten by the spirit.

NAPOLEON BONAPARTE

The Small Things in Daily Life

Do not think that love, in order to be genuine, has to be extraordinary. What we need is to love without getting tired.

How does a lamp burn? Through the continuous input of small drops of oil. ... My daughters, what are these drops of oil in our lamps? They are the small things of daily life: faithfulness, punctuality, small words of kindness, a thought for others, our way of being silent, of looking, of speaking, and of acting. These are the true drops of love ...

Be faithful in small things because it is in them that your strength lies.

MOTHER TERESA

8

Original goodness

The Self is divine.

The Self is at the core of every being as a lake is hidden in the mountains. Therefore, such attributes as kindness, compassion, and selflessness need not be learnt. They come from within. From the Self. They are already there. All that needs to be done is to clear the dirt that hides them.

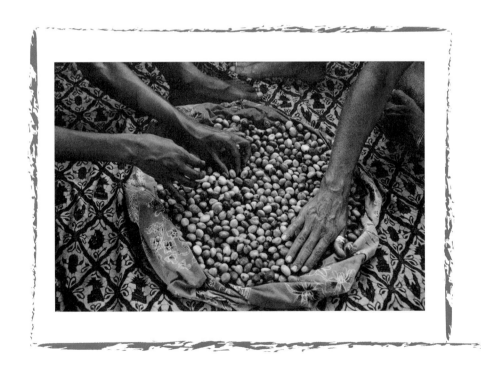

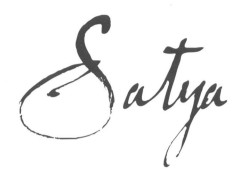

Satya

Truth

Satya is about bringing sincerity and integrity to all expressions.

It is about approaching the world with pure intentions.

It means to speak the truth with the spirit of kindness.

It means communicating from the heart.

Before you speak, ask yourself, is it kind, is it necessary, is it true,
does it improve on the silence?

SAI BABA

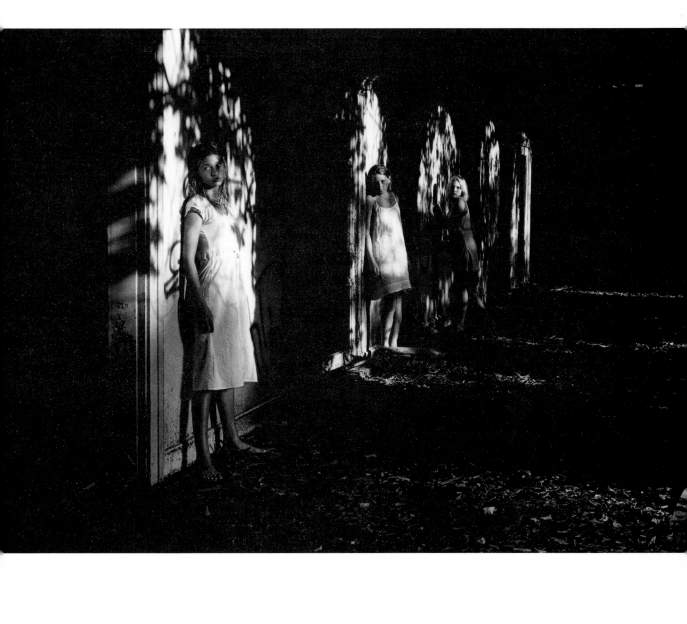

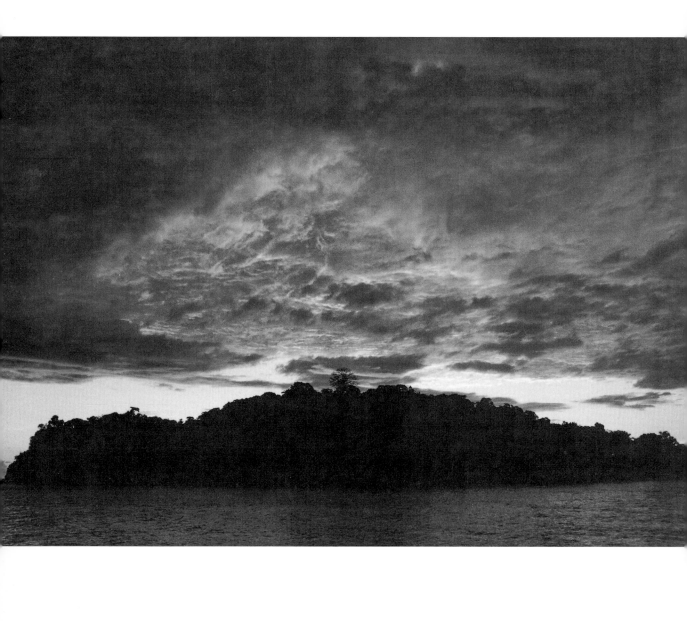

The Clear Blue Mind

— moral principles

Through the practice of *yama* you learn to go into the mind.

At first it is difficult to see clearly—your thoughts are so tightly stuck together. Like thick clouds in the sky.

Yama—the cool wind of clarity blows through. The clouds part. Dissolve. The sky lightens.

Your thoughts, still present, are now visible as themselves and not just as a tangled mass. You can see the outline of each cloud, its shape, texture, and mood.

When this starts to happen, you begin to sense the clear blue sky. The light of your true Self.

Asteya

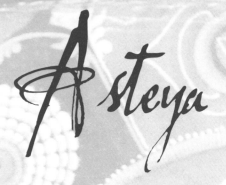

Non-stealing

Give up wanting what other people have.

RUMI

More than non-stealing.
Only taking what is freely given.
Only taking what we need.

Living simply.

The secret waits for eyes unclouded by longing.

LAO-TZU

Tao-Te-Ching

Expressed as a positive, *asteya* means generosity: to give, to share, and to rejoice.

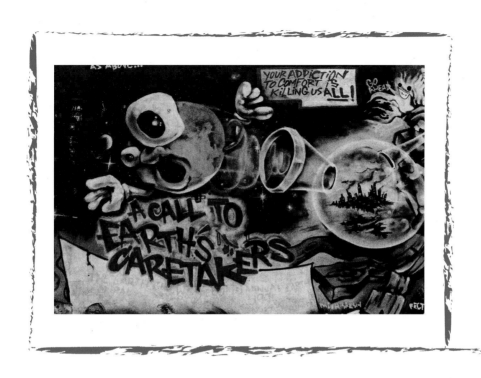

When one abstains from stealing, precious jewels shower down ...

PATANJALI

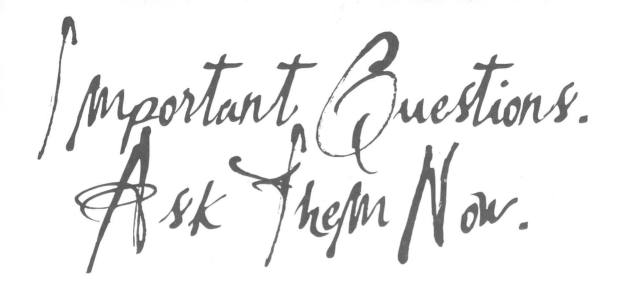

Important Questions. Ask Them Now.

In the whirlwind of our complex lives we can forget our deepest values and intentions. But when we come to the end of our lives and look back, what will we ask? What will have mattered most?

Did I win all my fights?

Did I make lots of money?

Did I make people see things my way?

Or will we ask

Did I live a full life?

Did I live with integrity?

Did I love well?

Most people die with their music still locked inside them.

BENJAMIN DISRAELI

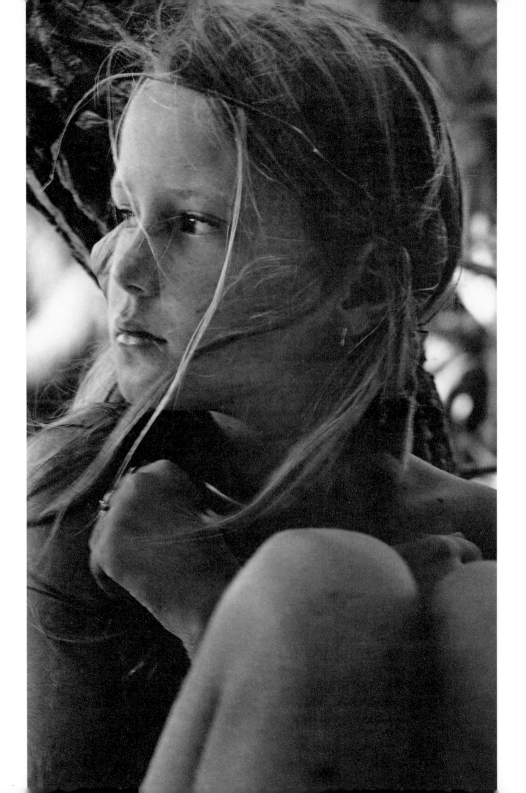

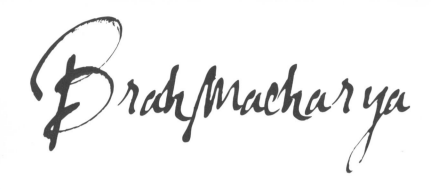

Brahmacharya

Commitment to the containment and harnessing of a primal force—sexuality

Sexual energy is one of the strongest forces in humans, and like any great power, it can be put to constructive or destructive use. It is the force that must be worked with, and gently trained so that it does not rule our minds and senses. Containment of sexuality is not about ruining your sex life. It is about transforming this vital force to a spiritual level. This redirection of energy will increase your inner strength and recharge depleted energy reserves.

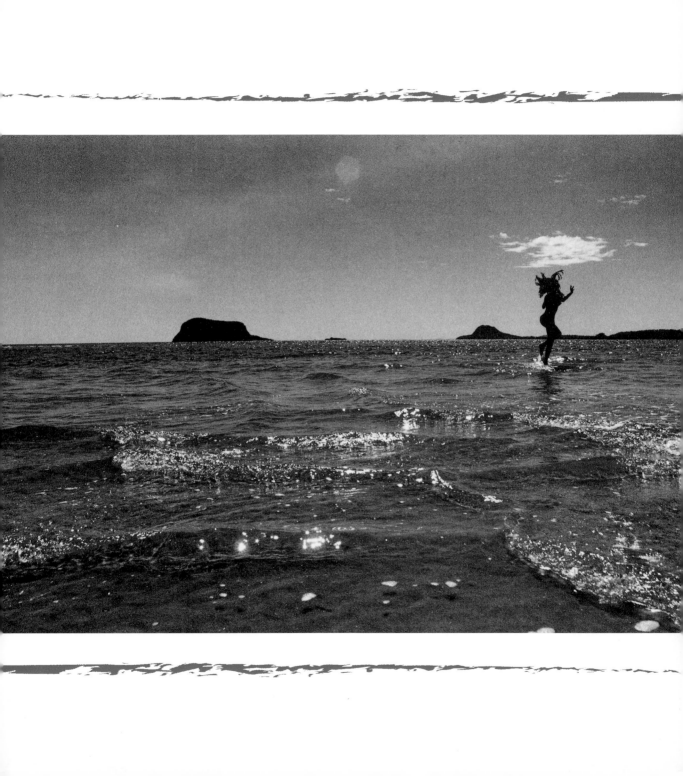

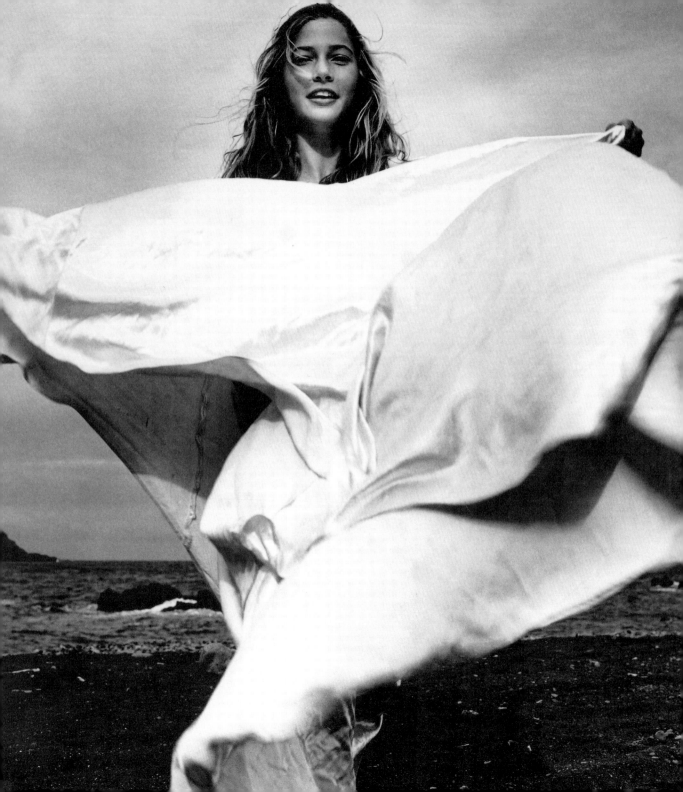

Do I contradict myself?

Very well, then I contradict myself.

I am large, I contain multitudes.

WALT WHITMAN

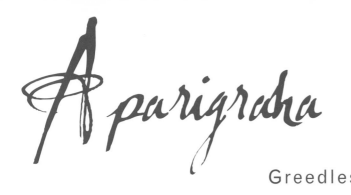

Aparigraha

Greedlessness

Whatever you have, you want more.

Wherever you are, you want to be somewhere else.

If you have straight hair, you want curly hair.

Breaking the infinite cycle of

Want ... Have ... Need

More

More

More

Never enough

I want to swallow the world

Stepping back. Watching and observing what you grasp for. Seeing beyond the small world of our personal desires. This is the fifth pillar of *yama*.

The world has enough for everyone's need, but not enough for everyone's greed.

GANDHI

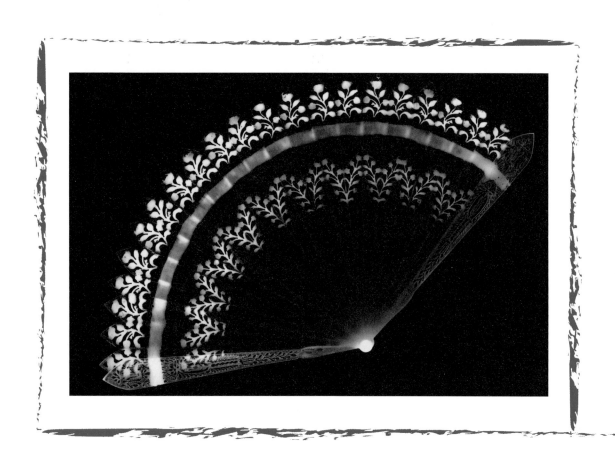

Give up wanting what other people have.

RUMI

Remember.

There is no joy without sorrow.

No good without bad.

No truth without lies.

As you begin your practice of *yama* do not be disturbed by what is unveiled.

Appreciate your flaws as you appreciate your qualities. They help you to learn.

We should find perfect existence through imperfect existence.

SHUNRYU SUZUKI

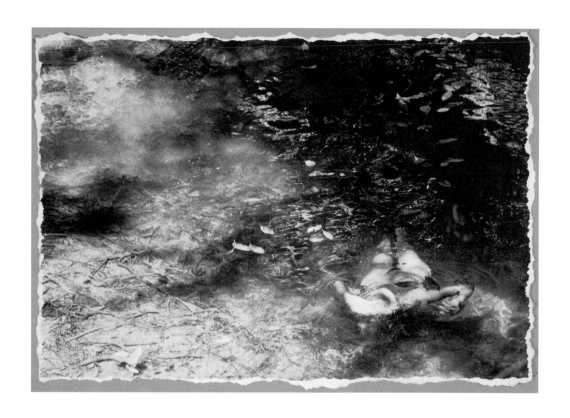

Do you have the patience to wait

Till your mud settles and the water is clear?

Can you remain unmoving

Till the right action arises by itself?

LAO-TZU

Tao-Te-Ching

The Ongoing Practice of Yama

When we begin the practice of *yama* our minds
are like puppies—jumpy and playful. But in time,
as our practice evolves and our mind is gently
trained, we become more attuned to the
subtleties of existence. When this happens, the
moral restraint of *yama* begins to emerge
naturally from within.

As our innate morality is awakened, it begins to
speak to us—a sort of echo, feeling,
reverberation. An in-your-gut, feels-good/
feels-bad type of knowledge.

Cultivate your inner senses. Listen. Reach in
through the muck. Cut the vines, the thorns.
Clear a pathway. Make a space for this inner
sound voice thing. Explore the subtle world.

26

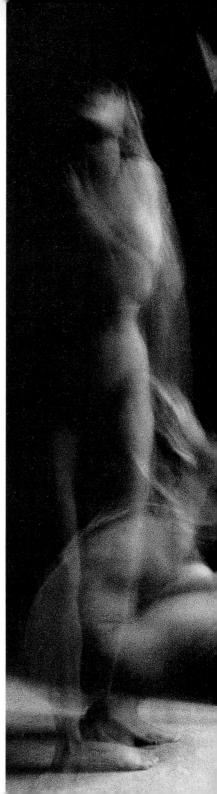

Niyama

Personal Disciplines

Yoga is skill in action

The Bhagavad Gita (II.50)

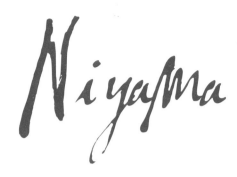

Niyama

Niyama is the second limb of the eightfold path of yoga. It is made up of five observances that are concerned with personal disciplines. They work on the ways that we approach ourselves.

Saucha	Purity
Santosha	Contentment
Tapas	Self-discipline
Svadhyaya	Self-study
Ishvara-pranidhana	Surrender

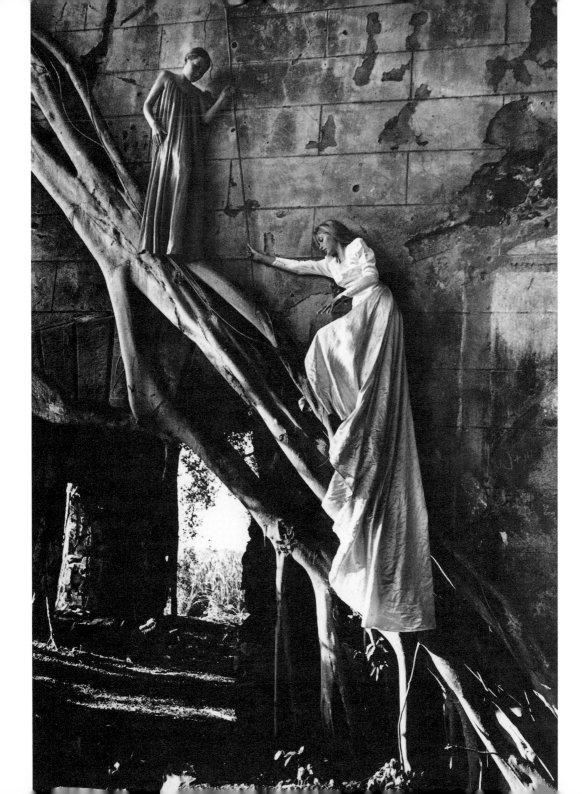

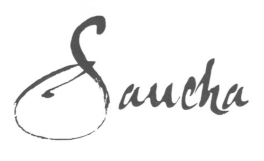Saucha

Purity

Engage in things that are purifying.

> Stretch.
>
> Breathe.
>
> Be aware.
>
> Be sincere.

We can practice purity in the way we select, prepare, and eat our food.

We can practice purity in conversation.

We can practice purity in thought.

Saucha, like all practices of the eightfold path, is experienced on different levels. For instance, taking a bath is an act of external cleansing. *Saucha* can take a physically cleansing form such as *asanas*, the physical postures of yoga. It can equally take on a spiritual dimension, such as happens after deep and prolonged meditation.

The entire search for our true essence is a process of purification and letting go. As the impurities dissolve, the light of self-knowledge and awareness emerges. The energy of the universe circulates freely.

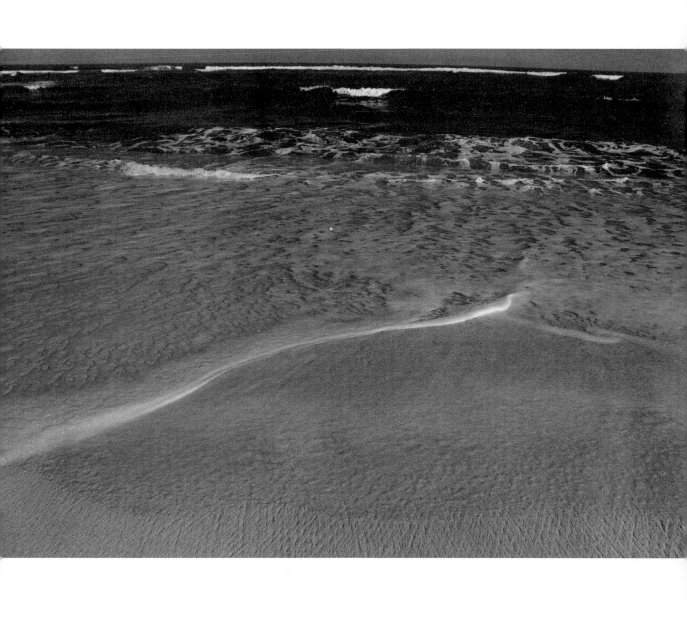

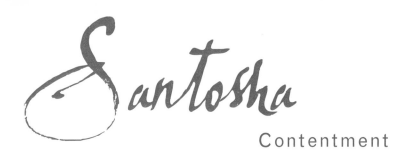

Santosha

Contentment

Acceptance of all that encompasses our lives.

Cultivating equanimity.

Wanting nothing = lacking nothing.

Dispassion.

Natural contentment arises.

This is *santosha*.

Dispassion/*vairagya*—not being the tennis ball in an eternal game between pleasure and pain, attachment, and aversion dictated by our mind and senses. Dispassion frees the spirit. It is not about being cold or cut off. It is simply a redirection of passion from the material world to the subtle world.

Acceptance—a graceful power. Accepting a situation, yet working to change it; accepting others yet still having choices about our relationship to them.

From contentment results unparalleled happiness.

PATANJALI

The real world is beyond our thoughts and ideas; we see it through the net of
our desires, divided into pleasure and pain, right and wrong, inner and outer.
To see the universe as it is, you must step beyond the net.
It is not hard to do so, for the net is full of holes.

SRI NISARGADATTA

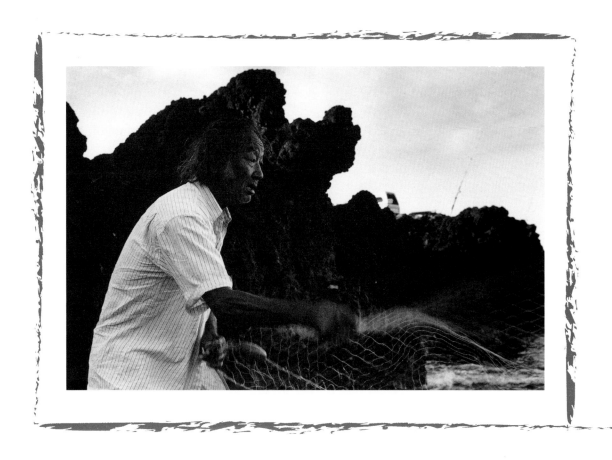

Actionless Action

Actionless action—working without any undercurrents of desire—is crucial to the path of yoga.

Why? Because when we mentally involve the ego in the things that we do, our desires and expectations create more entanglement with the world. We are pulled here and there by joy, by disappointment; unstable within ourselves. On the other hand, when we work selflessly, the mind stays pure. Whilst we are not indifferent to the result of our actions, we are not addicted to its fruits. Actionless action is a slow but important process of learning to rely on the strength and equanimity that comes from within. From the Self.

All of our desires for the fruits of life are caused
by a feeling of emptiness. Once we are genuinely
full, what other fruits could we desire?

Abhinavagupta

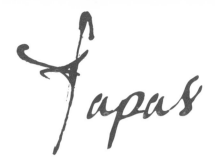

Self-discipline

Tapas is the conscious commitment to your aim. It is about devoting as much of your life as possible to that inner fire; the fire that illuminates the way and burns through all desires and obstacles.

Tapas is a way of expressing the passion in your heart.

P.S.

Tapas may cause tears but it should not cause suffering.

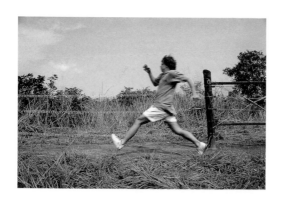

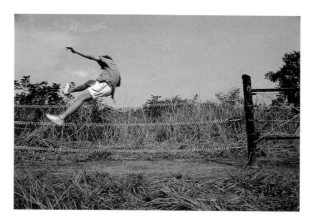

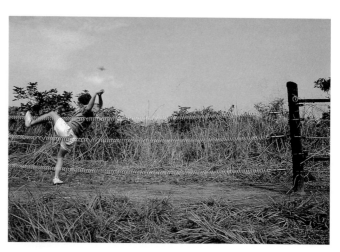

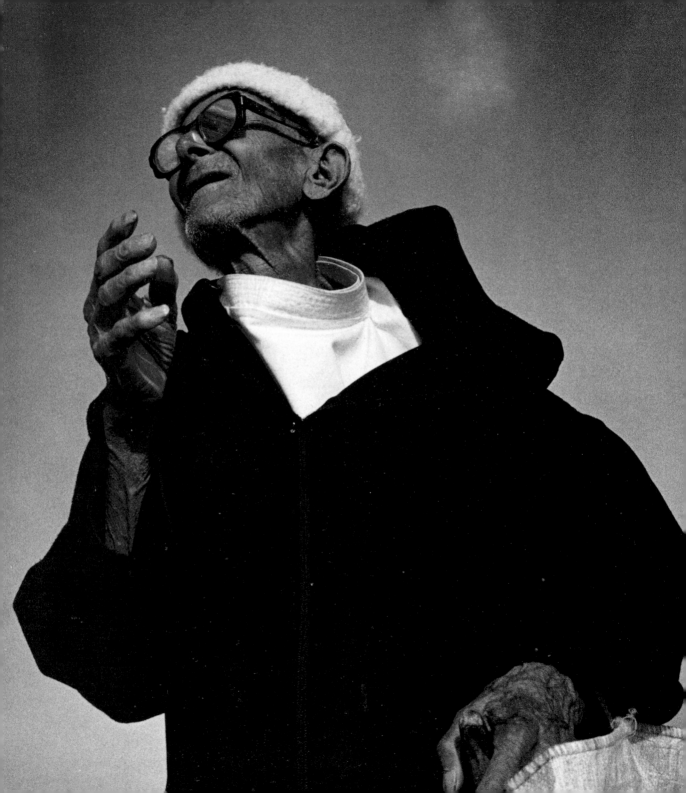

The World

A man from a town of Negua, on the coast of
Colombia, could climb into the sky.

On his return, he described his trip. He told how
he had contemplated human life from on high.
He said we are a sea of tiny flames.

Each person shines with his or her own light.
No two flames are alike. There are big flames and
little flames, flames of every color. Some people's
flames are so still they don't even flicker in the
wind while others have wild flames that fill the air
with sparks. Some foolish flames neither burn nor
shed light, but others blaze with life so fiercely
that you can't look at them without blinking and if
you approach, you shine in fire.

EDUARDO GALEANO

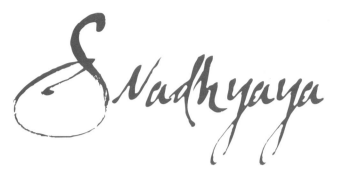

Svadhyaya

Self-study

Sva means "self ... belonging to me."

Adhyaya means "inquiring ... examination of something to get close to it."

Think of your com pu ter   A machine   A tool

with so   much

potential.

You can't use it if you don't get to know it.

Humans are similar.

We need to study ourselves.

We need to know our complexities, limitations, and potentials to best navigate the cables and conduits of life.

The longing to scratch the surface, to sniff, to search ...

The longing to understand.

Man did not weave the web of life: he is merely a strand in it.

Whatever he does to the web, he does to himself.

JIMMY GOLDSMITH

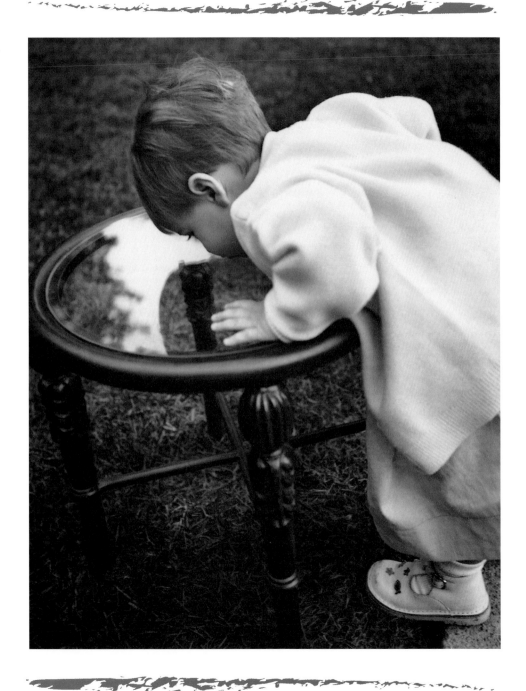

My life is not this steeply sloping hour,

in which you see me hurrying.

Much stands behind me; I stand before it like a tree;

I am only one of my many mouths

and at that, the one that will be still the soonest.

I am the rest between two notes,

which are somehow always in discord

because death's note wants to climb over –

but in the dark interval, reconciled,

they stay there trembling.

    And the song goes on, beautiful.

RAINER MARIA RILKE

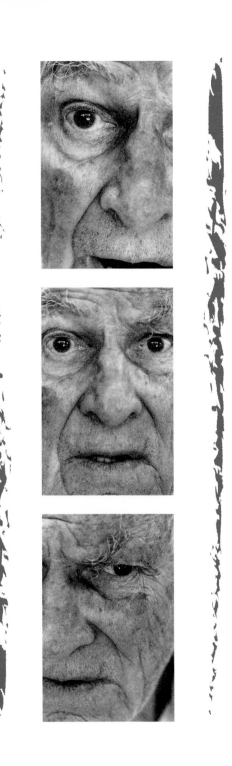

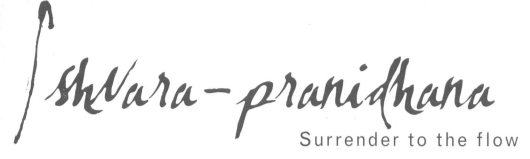

Ishvara-pranidhana

Surrender to the flow

TO TAKE SHELTER IN THE SUPREME

Letting go.

Trusting.

A joyful surrender.

Offering the fruits of your actions to a higher purpose.

Spirituality becomes the point and purpose of our lives.

The attainment of wholeness requires one to stake one's whole being.
Nothing less will do; there can be no easier conditions,
no substitutes, no compromises.

C. G. JUNG

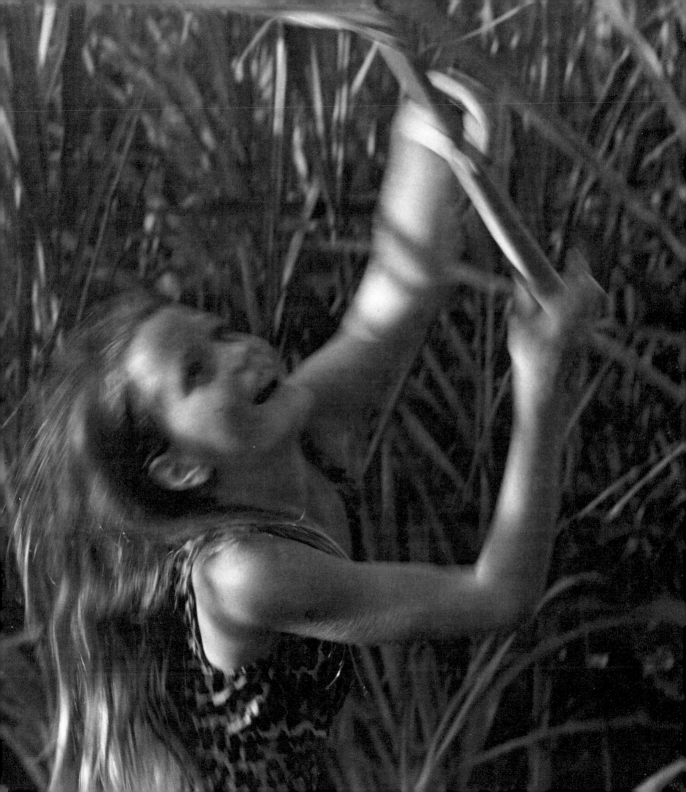

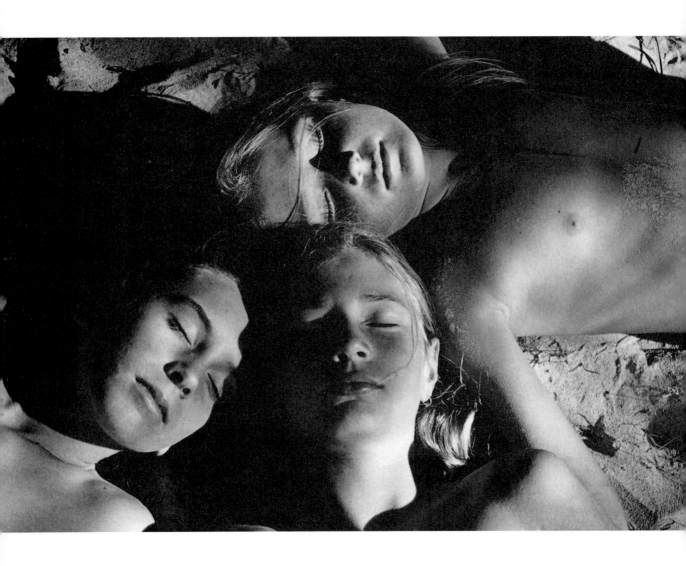

The direct practice of *yama* and *niyama* may result in frustration.

Yoga is not about frustration.

Create time to be still.

This brings us to our center.

Whether we are able to feel it or not, it connects us to our core.

In this core *yama* and *niyama* exist naturally.

They are part of your natural morality.

The more you sift through the clutter, the more space you give for your natural purity to emerge. And eventually the practice of *yama* and *niyama* will no longer be an exterior source of guidance.

They will come from within. Spontaneously.

They will come from you.

The search may begin with a restless feeling, as if one were being watched. One turns in all directions and sees nothing. Yet one senses that there is a source for this deep restlessness; and the path that leads there is not a path to a strange place, but the path home. ("But you *are* home," cries the Witch of the North. "All you have to do is wake up!") The journey is hard, for the secret place *where we have always been* is overgrown with thorns and thickets of "ideas," of fears and defenses, prejudices and repressions. The holy grail is what Zen Buddhists call our own "true nature;" each man is his own savior after all.

PETER MATTHIESSEN
The Snow Leopard

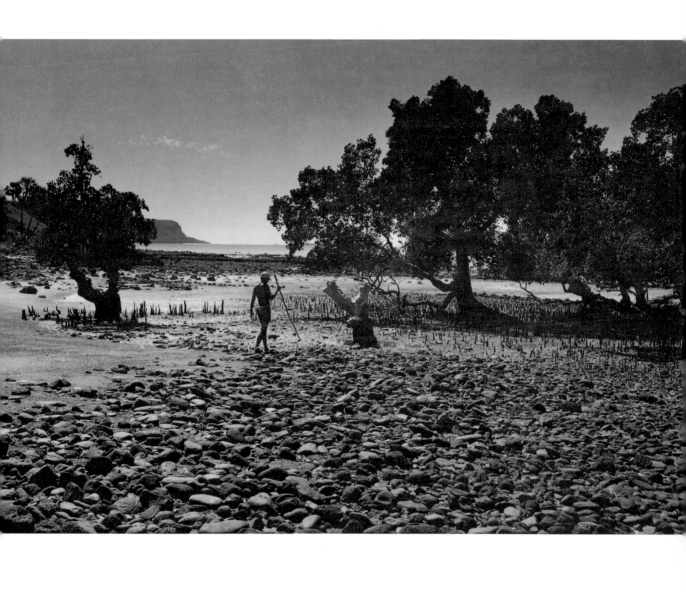

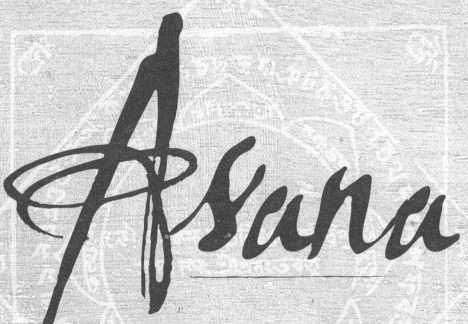

Asana

Physical Postures

You asked me what I came into the world to do.

I came to live out loud.

EMILE ZOLA

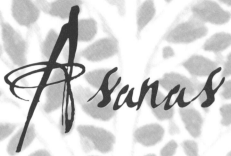

Asanas

The Postures of Yoga

Asana is the third limb of Patanjali's sutras, and the gate through which most westerners enter yoga practice.

Asanas are the physical postures of yoga. Ancient, tried-and-tested exercises, developed over thousands of years to purposefully exercise every muscle, nerve, and gland in the human body.

A committed practice of *asanas* will make the body strong yet elastic, light yet grounded. No equipment is needed. Just you, your determination, the mat, and the breath.

Asanas are a gateway to the Self: they train the body and focus the mind, making it a fit vehicle for the soul.

The Sea

Stroke by
   stroke my
      body remembers that life and cries for
      the lost parts of itself –
fins, gills
   opening like flowers into
      the flesh – my legs
      want to lock and become
one muscle, I swear I know
   just what the blue-gray scales
      shingling
      the rest of me would
feel like!
   paradise! Sprawled
      in the motherlap
      in that dreamhouse
of salt and exercise,
   what a spillage
      of nostalgia pleads
      from the very bones! how
they long to give up the long trek
   inland, the brittle
      beauty of understanding,
      and dive,
and simply
   become again a flaming body
      of blind feeling
      slinking along
in the luminous roughage of the sea's body,
   vanished
      like victory inside that
      insucking genesis, that
roaring flamboyance, that
   perfect
      beginning and
      conclusion of our own.

MARY OLIVER

Why Practice Asanas?

Asanas work on many different levels.

At first our bodies solely feel the outward physical experience of
this practice.
Every pose seems torturous.
Our bodies trembling, sweaty, and exhausted.

Then, at some point, it becomes a necessity. The blissful lengthening and
strengthening of muscle, skin, and flesh. And the quality of your mind …
cleansed, refreshed, calm. It is a practice that anchors you. It helps you live
in a more positive and less chaotic fashion. People close to you notice
the difference.

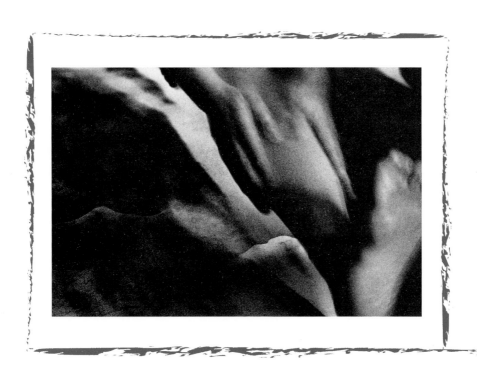

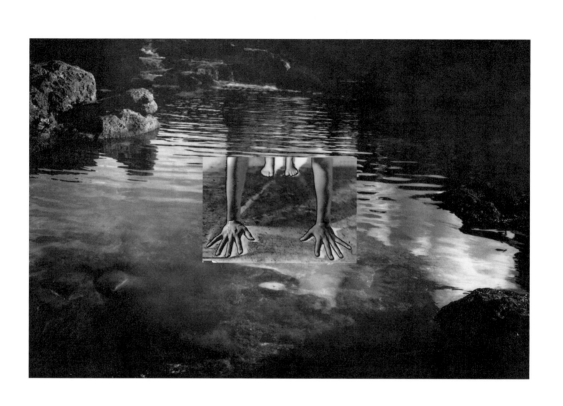

Asanas are not just stretching exercises. They are a feeling—an exploration of Self.

The practice of *asanas* invites us to direct our mind and breath to the core of each posture, helping to open locked areas and release imbalances that prevent the body from being in correct alignment. This tremendous harnessing of our faculties draws us deeper and deeper through the layers of our being.

As we become more and more settled in the core of each posture, the dualities between body and mind, mind and soul begin to dissolve. An inner awareness and subtlety evolves, and the *asana* becomes a state of being in itself.

When the posture of yoga is steady and easy, resting like the cosmic serpent on the waters of infinity. Then one is unconstrained by opposing dualities.

PATANJALI

The Ritual of Practice

The moment you unroll your mat you are entering a disciplined practice. Honor it as such.

Begin each practice by sitting or standing for a few minutes in silence. This creates a psychological break from the concerns of everyday life and helps to bring the focus and intent necessary to complete your practice.

Always end by resting the body in *shavasana*. This allows the effects of your practice to settle peacefully in the body. It is also a time to refresh the mind by letting go and slipping out of mind-talk. The practice of *asanas* will have quieted the mind. *Shavasana*, or rest pose, is the time to enjoy this effect.

When leaving *shavasana*, gently roll over to one side and wait a few moments before opening your eyes to allow the body and mind to adjust to the "real" world. Bring care and attention when rolling up your mat, keeping your focus alive until the very end. Eventually this focus will start to flow out of your practice and into your life.

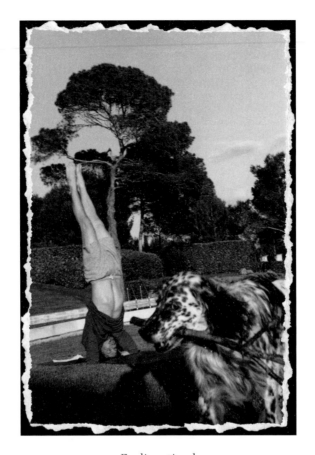

Feeling tired.

Not in the mood.

Your body's aching.

Stiff.

You've got other things to do.

Can't slow your mind down.

Just get on the mat.

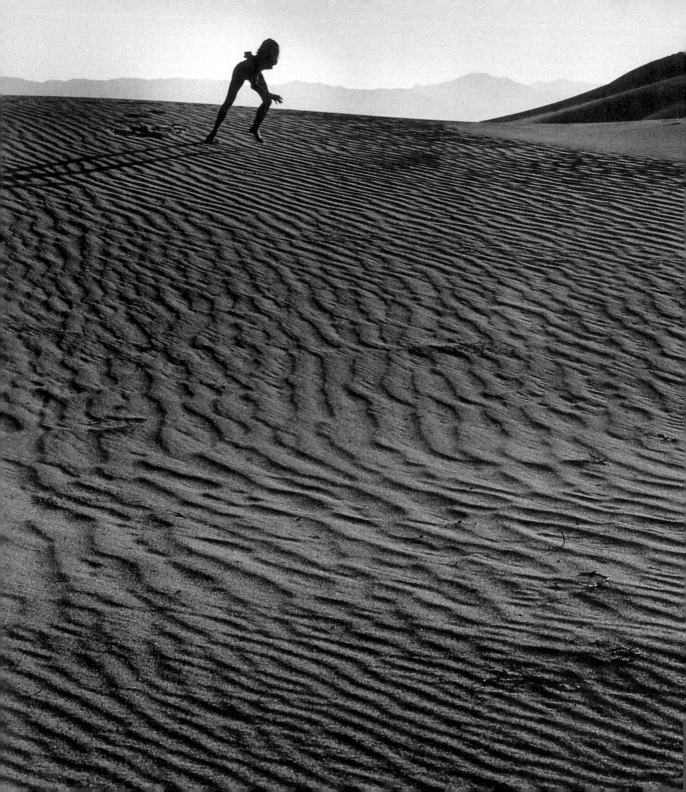

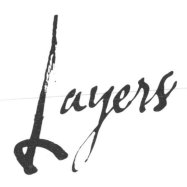

Layers

Asanas teach us to pay attention. To focus. To concentrate.

If we don't, we put our bodies at risk. We get injured.

The more we practice this engagement, the more natural it becomes.

It's about layers.

Adding gentle layer upon layer.

Opening layer below layer.

Reaching a different space.

What is Yoga?

Space in my body.

MOTHER

Meditation for Tadasana

Stand with your feet together, tailbone tucked, and sternum lifted.

Bring your attention to the feet.

Feel them broad, spread, and full.

Press down powerfully through the heels until you feel the

earth pushing back up.

Let this push expand upwards through the shin bones, the front thighs,

and into the torso.

Draw your muscles up through the body.

Feel how they lengthen, open, change shape.

Grow into the space above your head.

Imagine a string attached to the crown of your head.

It gently lifts you as you keep pushing down.

While keeping the body strong, soften the inner ears.

Think of your lower jaw full of water.

Let this water trickle down your organs melting tightness in the throat,

the heart, the stomach.

Continue to soften internally, but keep the physical shell strong and stable.

Think of your tailbone uncurling like a fern.

Feel yourself rooted.

Stay open.

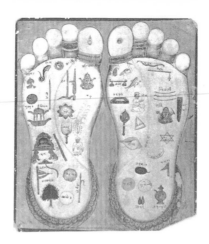

The heavy is the root of light.
The unmoved is the source of all movement.

Thus the master travels all day
without leaving home.
However splendid the views,
she stays serenely in herself.

Why should the lord of the country
flit about like a fool?
If you let yourself be blown to and fro,
you lose touch with your root.
If you let restlessness move you,
you lose touch with who you are.

LAO-TZU
Tao-Te-Ching

Surya Namaskara

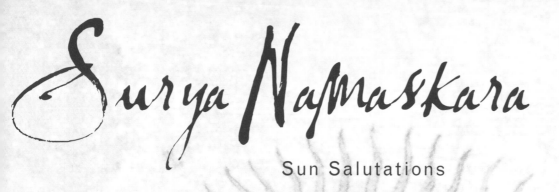

Sun Salutations

By steady concentration, contemplation, and dissolution

with the sun, one has knowledge of the worlds.

PATANJALI

Sun salutations are a powerful combination of *asanas*, which have been linked together to form a sequence in themselves. Although the technique can vary, the flow of the sequence remains the same. It moves in and out of forward and backward bends, stretching, revitalizing and toning the entire body, from the tips of the hands to the tips of the feet.

Sun salutations can be used to generate strong internal heat and give a good stretch to the body. They make the spine supple and youthful, releasing deep tension.

This magical sequence of postures can serve as a powerful link between poses. It can also be a practice in itself.

In one salutation to thee, my God, let all my senses spread out
and touch this world at thy feet.

Like a rain-cloud of July hung low with its burden of unshed showers let
all my mind bend down at thy door in one salutation to thee.

Let all my songs gather together their diverse strains into a single current
and flow to a sea of silence in one salutation to thee.

Like a flock of homesick cranes flying day and night back to their mountain
nests let all my life take its voyage to its eternal home in one salutation to thee.

RABINDRANATH TAGORE
Gitanjali (Song Offerings)

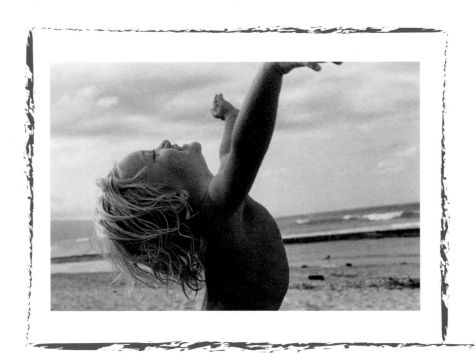

Standing Poses

The Back Leg

Always maintain awareness of the back leg in all standing poses. The back leg is your foundation, your strength, your structure. When commitment and intensity are absent from the back leg, the pose as a whole will not evolve.

As I dig for wild orchids
in the autumn fields,
it is the deeply bedded root
that I desire,
not the flower.

IZUMI SHIKIBU

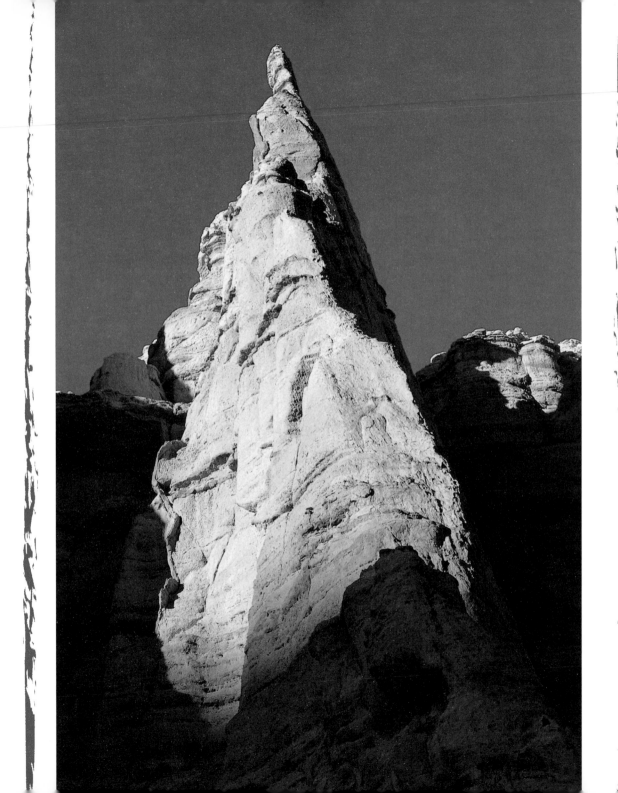

The Hands

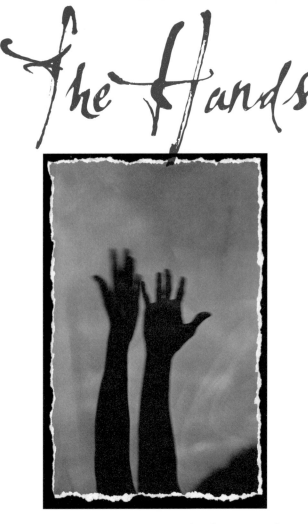

Extend the energy in your body outwards.

Feel it coursing through the elbows, the wrist, the warm palms of the hands
To each finger tip and beyond …

Remember your hands. Keep them alive.
Engage to your full potential.

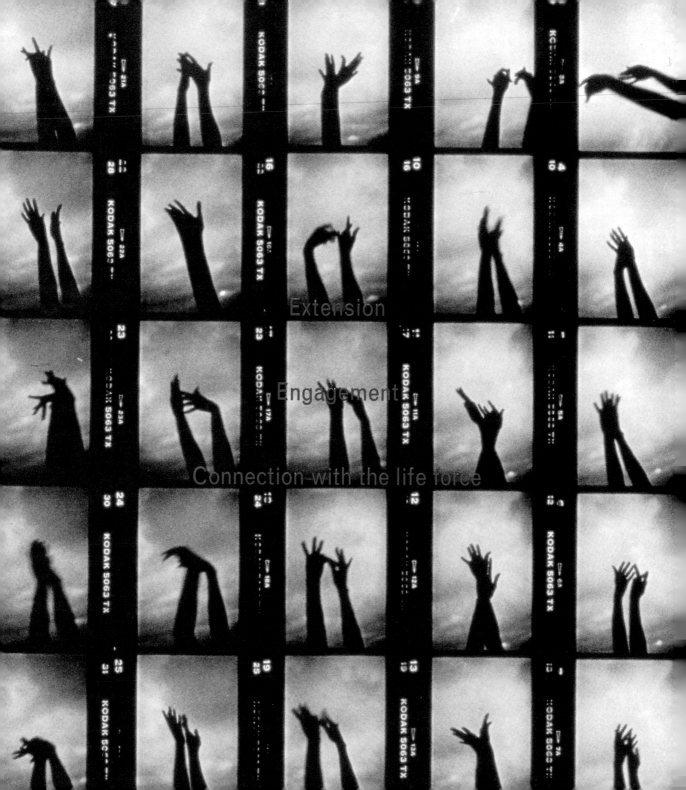

Extension

Engagement

Connection with the life force

Seated Twists

Twists work in many ways. For instance, they adjust the spine, tone the spinal nerves, and ease stomach ailments by stretching the inner digestive organs. They are also wonderful detoxifiers as they wring the old blood from the spine, recharging it with fresh sustenance.

When twisting, bring your inner eye into your spine, the vertical axis of the body. Press your sitbones down, rooting them firmly into the earth, and work your attention upwards from the base, vertebrae by vertebrae. Keep the spine long while twisting from your center—from the root. Use each inhale to lengthen the spine and each exhale to deepen the twisting motion. Be a corkscrew.

Remember that, like any *asana*, a twist involves holding the structure of the pose while softening the internal body within this structure. In other words, holding the vertical axis of your spine but softening around it. This softening is what will help to deepen your pose more than pulling and pushing. The movement must come from within. The flesh, muscles, and cells must release their tight grip. Each time you twist, become conscious of this cleansing and releasing process. Rejoice in it.

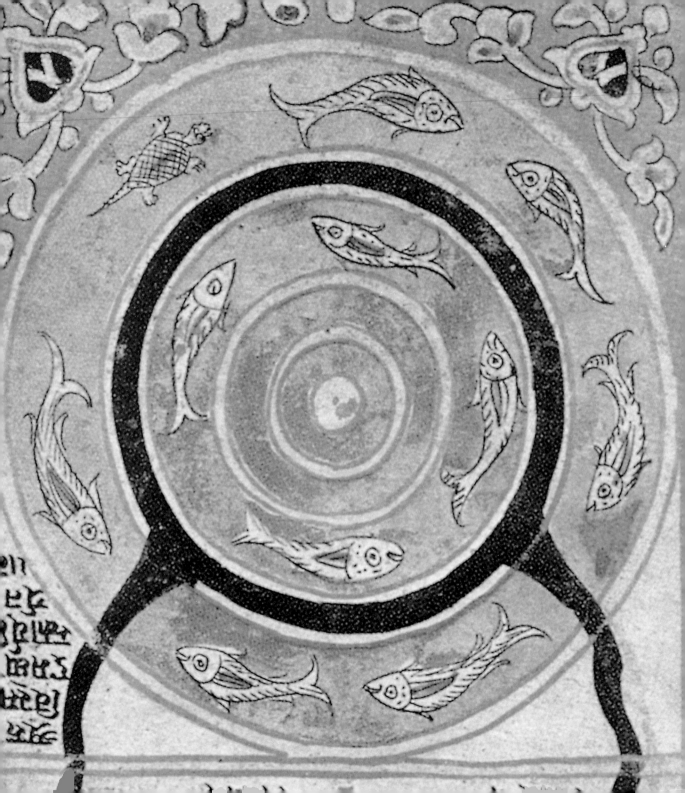

Inversions

Inversions are the royal poses of yoga, revered since ancient times for their remarkable restorative and revitalizing effects.

In *shirshasana*, or headstand, the reversal of the body's gravity brings a fresh supply of healthy blood to the head and chest, the seat of power, knowledge, intelligence and breath. Brain cells are bathed and nourished, and the mind is revived. With continued practice, thinking becomes clearer, sleep and memory are improved, headaches disappear.

In *sarvangasana*, or shoulderstand, rich blood flows to the chest and neck areas, relieving common ailments such as colds and asthma, and to the abdominal organs, easing the digestive system and relieving menstrual problems.

Nerves are soothed.

Toxins are freed.

New life flows.

Vitality is restored.

Life is normally viewed with our bodies the right way up.

With inversions our world is turned upside down.

Eyes now at ground level.

A new perspective.

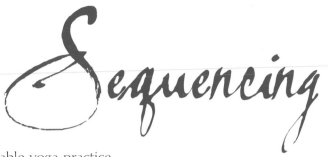

Sequencing

Structure is the secret to an enjoyable yoga practice.

Asanas cannot be jumbled together any which way. The proper sequencing of poses is crucial to the effective opening and closing of the body. Each posture has a specific effect on the body. When combined with another posture, these effects can be used to heal, raise energetic states, soothe … It is powerful stuff.

The proper combination of *asanas* is crucial to an intelligent understanding of yoga that goes beyond mere repetition of postures.

Yoga is an art and a science. The sequencing of *asanas* is the science of yoga.

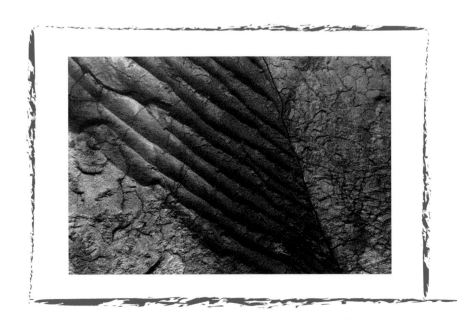

Think of your body as two bodies working together. You have the outer physical shell and an inner soft pulsing energy body. Most of us have locked the energy body inside our skeletal shell. We can do this without meaning to. Anger, disappointment, stress … all the things we experience on a day-to-day basis accumulate in our physiques. Although this inner body continues to subtly feed your outer body, it is trapped and weak. It cannot move, be heard or express itself.

The practice of *asanas* awakens the intelligence of this inner body. It is as if the cells emerge from hibernation and begin to communicate with each other again. When this takes place you enter a deeper layer of practice and awareness. Poses that initially seemed simple reveal themselves as complex. You feel the need to slow down and explore postures, feeling the body from the inside out.

This inner body of energy is impossible to ignore once it finds its voice. It speaks to you, calls you, teaches you, and gives you a sense of the power beyond. The power of your inner oasis, the power of your true Self begins to emerge.

I Talk to My Body

My body, you are an animal
whose appropriate behavior
is concentration and discipline.
An effort
of an athlete, of a saint and of a yogi.

Well trained
you may become for me
a gate
through which I will leave myself
and a gate
through which I will enter myself.
A plumb line to the center of the earth
and a cosmic ship to Jupiter.

My body, you are an animal
for whom ambition
is right.
Splendid possibilities
are open to us.

ANNA SWIR

Whilst technique in an *asana* is, of course, crucial, it is just as important to create *bahava*—mood—in your practice.

Essentially yoga is a state of existence, and *bahava* is the color, taste, smell, and feel of this experience. *Bahava* comes from inspiration. It is a gift. It will permeate your being more strongly than the most precise instructions.

The Silence

Listen my child, to the silence.

An unknowing silence,

a silence

that turns valleys and echoes slippery,

bends foreheads

toward the ground.

FEDERICO GARCÍA LORCA

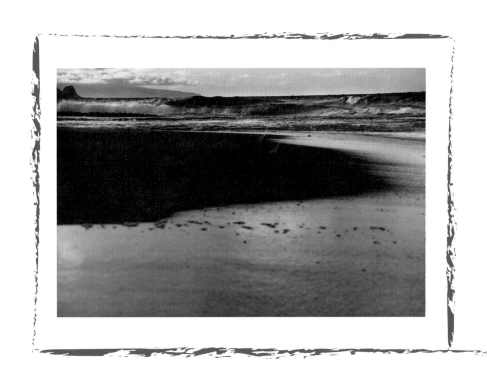

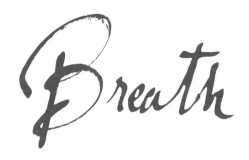

Breath

Most of the time we are not aware of our breath. The practice of *asanas* forces us to start noticing how we breathe. Is the breath smooth or ragged? Are the inhales and exhales long or short? Do we breathe from our noses or our mouths? Perhaps it changes all the time.

As you become aware of the quality of your breath you will begin to notice how you experience it in your body. Are you breathing from your belly or your chest? What does the breath come in contact with while it completes a cycle of inhale and exhale? Do you feel yourself expanding, widening, opening?

The breath is a key to unlocking your body and deepening your practice. Allow yourself to *feel* the pose through your breath. Let it slide over muscles, through sinew, breeze over joints. Follow the evanescent trail.

When you can actively use the breath as a tool to enter a deeper state of awareness in any posture, your *asana* practice will radically change. It will flow. It will be smooth. It will energize, and it will also calm your entire being.

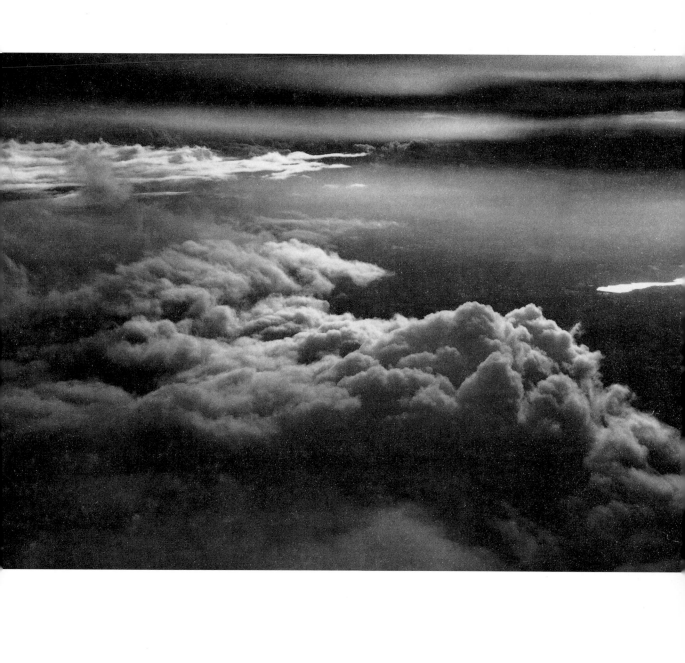

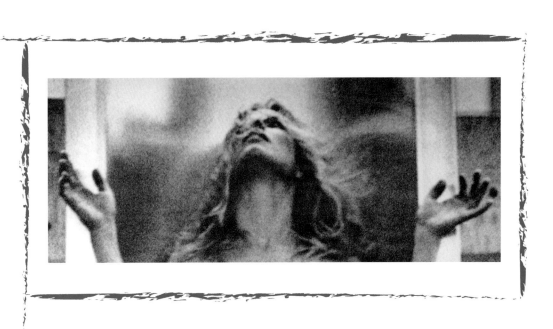

One of the benefits of a focused *asana* practice is that you start to become aware of the negative experiences stored in your body. Feelings of tightness and discomfort, hollow sensations, contractions, are all physical expressions of emotional states. The practice of *asanas* releases these blockages helping to make the body free-flowing. In making the body smooth and open the mind too becomes light … the sky of the mind becomes blue clear.

Where does the body end and the mind begin? Where does the mind end and the spirit begin? They cannot be divided as they are interrelated and but different aspects of the same all-pervading divine consciousness.

B. K. S. IYENGAR

Light on Yoga

So *asanas* slowly work to release physical tension and the deeper tensions that haunt the marrow of our bones.

New Blossoms of Me

The initial sense of renewal that you get from your yoga practice comes from the unleashing of inner energy that has been bound and locked—the energy of your true Self. Through the practice of *asanas* these restrictions, blocks, tensions, held deep within the cellular structure of the body are gradually released.

This unleashed dormant energy bubbles and flows. Like sap.

Bringing new growth.

Tender young buds.

New blossoms of you.

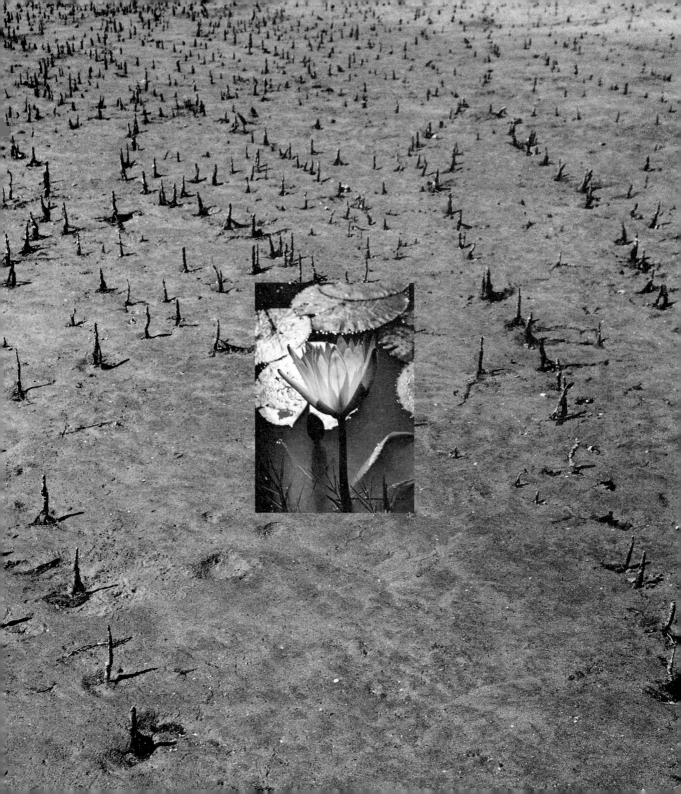

Yoga Diet

You need to eat food, but not all day long. It is the same thing with your practice of *asanas*. Use the state of mind created through your *asana* experience to sustain you until the next session. Just as it would be too much to expect one meal a week to keep you energized all week long, it is too much to expect one yoga class to do the same. In order to benefit from the light of yoga, you ultimately need to establish a regular daily practice.

Nourish yourself regularly and your energy will remain fluid, shiny, and clear.

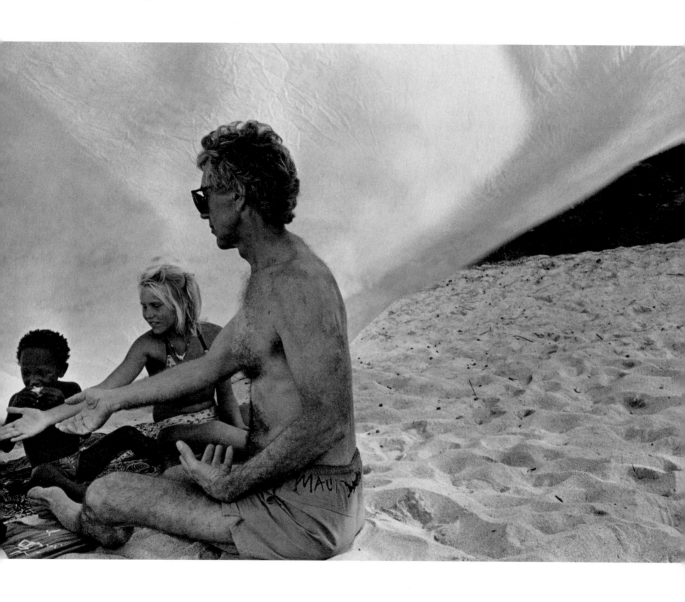

Compact as a Diamond

Yoga is a journey of energy discovery. Our own energy, the outside energy of the world ...

Scientifically speaking, energy travels most strongly through dense objects. The practice of *asanas* prepares the body for this by making it strong, compact, and robust. It slowly changes the body tissue, increasing the ratio of volume to weight, until the body is structurally heavy and dense.

Essentially *asanas* create a lightening rod out of our physiques, through which we gradually learn to control the electricity of the life-force—*prana*—with safety.

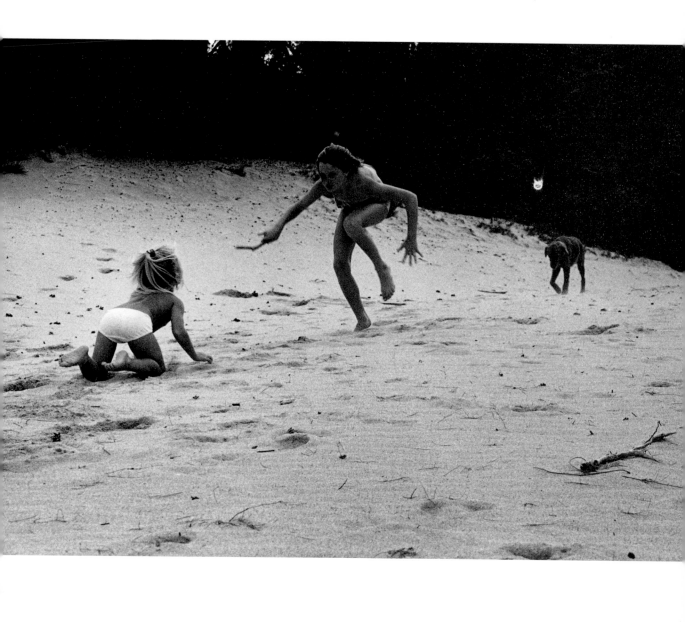

the experience of you in yourself

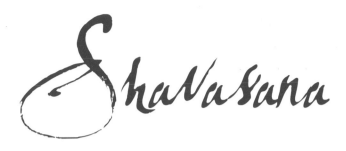

Shavasana, or rest pose, is an experience in itself.
It is the pose through which we discover softness.
It is the pose through which we dissolve into the earth.
It is the pose through which we begin to experience *pranayama*.
It is subtle and magical.
It is bliss.

Do not approach this posture as simple relaxation. It is an *asana* and, as such, is guided by specific boundaries within which we feel the experience.

When first starting an *asana* practice, it is often difficult to allow ourselves to rest enough to enter this pose. We tend to lie there thinking about the things we need to get done, and other such mind stuff.

For most people, it is easier to be active than to be passive.
Shavasana is the practice of active relaxation. It takes time to understand and experience, but it is deeply rewarding and refreshing.

It is a necessity to any *asana* practice as it gently seals the body's energy.

It is a cool swim in a green river.
It is the underwater sound of the ocean.
It is the soft pulsing coral at the bottom of the sea.

It is the experience of you in yourself. Dive deep.

Bridge to Our Inner World

Shavasana is a crucial link between *asanas* and *pranayama* because it teaches us to surrender in a passive state.

In order to bathe in the inner experience of *pranayama* we first need to be able to soften and open, both physically and mentally.

In *shavasana* this is what we learn to do. It is the posture in which we really let go of ourselves. It is a bridge to our inner world and inner energy. This so-called inner energy can actually be felt on a physical level as something inside our bodies. For some people it whirls, melts, prickles, heats, electrifies—but there is no denying its existence. The brain and heart pulse more slowly, the mind releases its hold on external issues, and something inside ourselves emerges. It is almost as if our inner Self steps forth, and our outer Self sits down and watches. Breathing in the ocean of grace.

Forgotten

Close your eyes and lose yourself in shadows
under the shadows of your eyelids' red-leaf forest.

Go down among those spirals
of sound humming and falling
and sounding faraway, remote,
all the way to the eardrum,
a deafened waterfall.

Send yourself down to the shadows,
drown yourself in your skin,
further, in your entrails:
let the bone, with its livid spark,
dazzle and blind you,
and among chasms and the gulfs of shadow
open its blue panache, will-o-wisp.

And in this liquid shadow of the dream
now bathe your nakedness;
relinquish your form, your foam
(nobody knows who flung it on the shore);
lose your self in your self, infinity
in your infinite being,
sea losing itself in another sea:
forget yourself and forget me.

In that forgetfulness ageless and endless
lips, kisses, love, all, born again:
the stars are daughters of night.

OCTAVIO PAZ

Pranayama

Breath Control

The whirlpools of the mind can be stilled by the breath.

PATANJALI

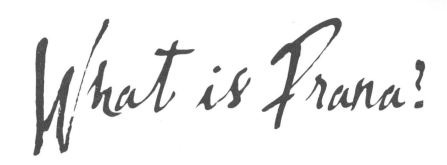

What is Prana?

It is as difficult to explain *prana* as it is to explain God.

B. K. S. IYENGAR

Prana is everything. It is everywhere.

It is the breath of the universe.

It is force, vitality.

It is creation. It is destruction.

It is life.

Prana burns as fire; he is the sun;

He is the beautiful rain god; he is the wind;

He is the earth, matter, God.

He is being and non-being and what is immortal.

Prashna Upanishad (II.5)

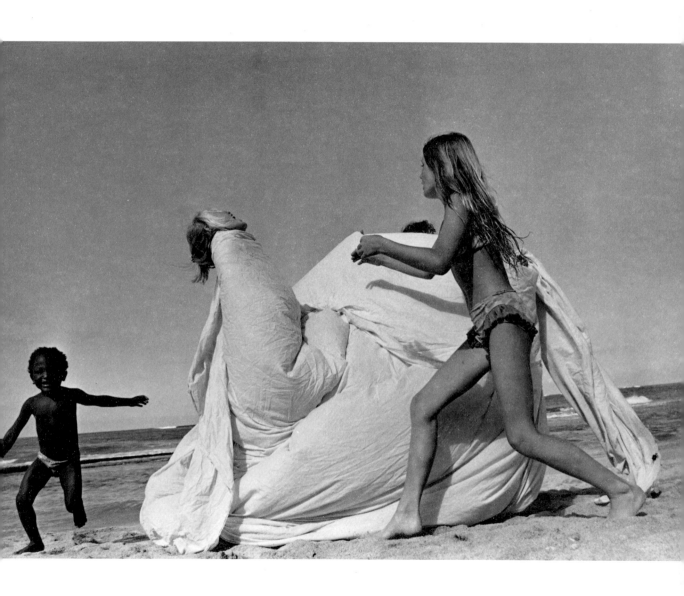

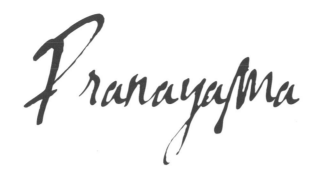

prana: life, energy, vitality

ayama: length, breadth, regulation, prolongation, control

Pranayama is the practice of regulating the flow of *prana* throughout the body using the breath.

Pranayama is essential. It is life giving. It is the practice that connects our inner energy with the outer energy. It is the way of controlling the vital force.

It is the art and science of discovering the soul.

> As long as there is breath in the body, there is life. When breath departs, so too does life. Therefore, practice *pranayama*.
>
> **SWAMI SVATMARAMA**
> *Hatha Yoga Pradipika* (2:3)

Purification through Pranayama

Prana has its own force, its own movement. It can never be completely controlled. All we can hope to do is create the ideal conditions within our body for *prana* to circulate and permeate its every crevice and shadow.

One of the main ways to facilitate this is through the cleansing and purification of the body. The less rubbish we have polluting us, the more *prana* can circulate.

Asanas work with the body to cleanse and open blockages. *Pranayama* uses the breath to purify on a deeper level. As the rubbish in our bodies is burnt and cleared away, *prana* will naturally flow by itself into the new clearings — filling us with the potent energy of life.

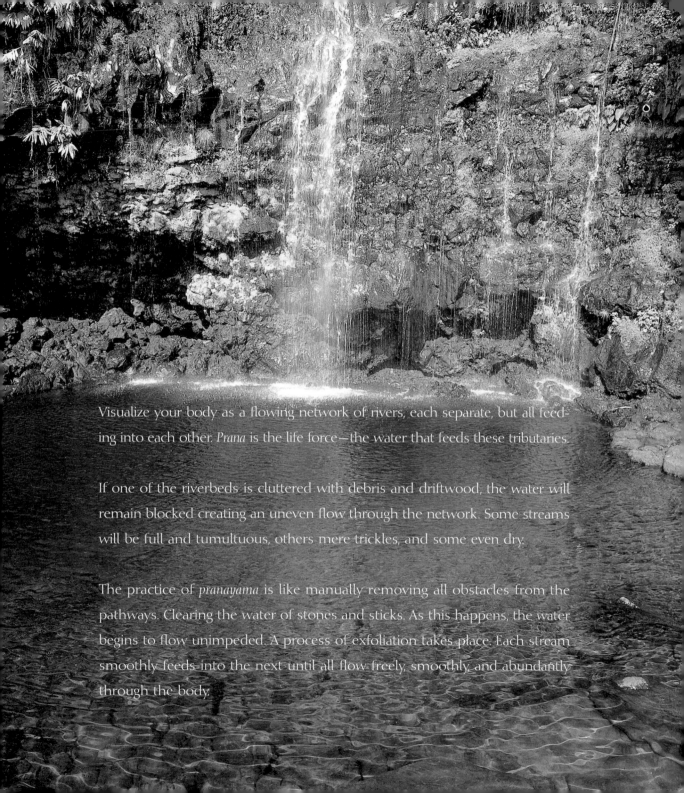

Visualize your body as a flowing network of rivers, each separate, but all feeding into each other. *Prana* is the life force—the water that feeds these tributaries.

If one of the riverbeds is cluttered with debris and driftwood, the water will remain blocked creating an uneven flow through the network. Some streams will be full and tumultuous, others mere trickles, and some even dry.

The practice of *pranayama* is like manually removing all obstacles from the pathways. Clearing the water of stones and sticks. As this happens, the water begins to flow unimpeded. A process of exfoliation takes place. Each stream smoothly feeds into the next until all flow freely, smoothly, and abundantly through the body.

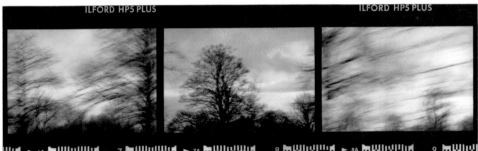

The Energetic World

While *pranayama* is the practice of controlling the flow of *prana* in the body, it is at the same time a way of resting the mind by engaging our attention in the breath. This focusing of the breath leads us to meditation and inner stillness. We slip out of the physical and into the ethereal world of the spirit.

As our practice of *pranayama* deepens, we start to feel inner vibrations, sensations, tinglings that we have not felt before. This is the energy of the outer world. Unlocking ourselves, we invite the world into us. We begin to recognize this other energy. We begin to let go of the I, the me me me.

Three Stages of Breath

> *Pranayama* is the regulation of the incoming and outgoing flow of breath with retention.
>
> PATANJALI

Inhalation
Puraka

Absorb the energy around you deep into your lungs, your blood, your tissue.

Retention
Kumbhaka

Let the outer breath mingle with the inner breath, the universal Self with the individual Self.

Exhalation
Rechaka

Feel yourself pouring into an infinite space. Trust. Give. Surrender to everything around you.

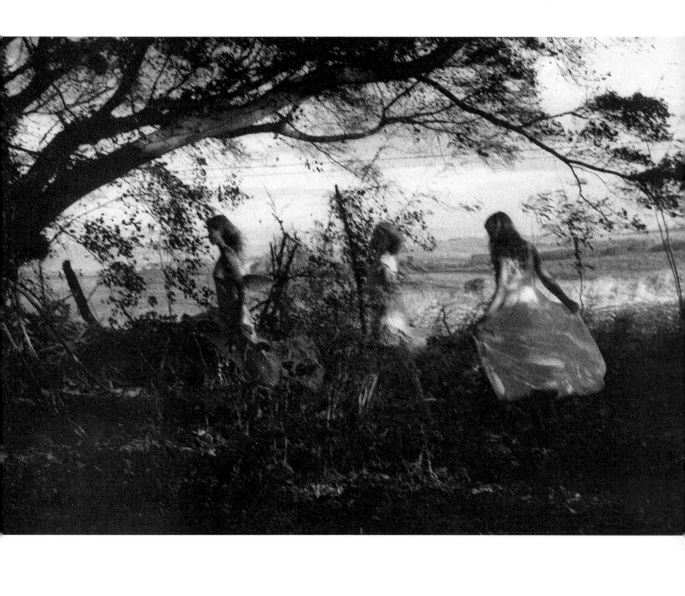

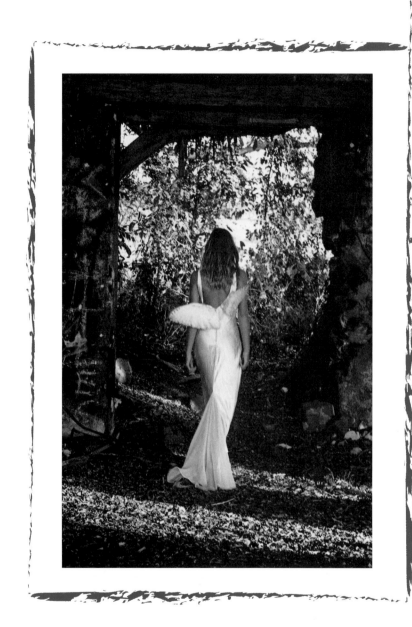

The distant shores of silence begin

at the door. You cannot fly there

like a bird. You must stop, look deeper

still deeper, until nothing deflects the soul

from the deepmost deep.

KAROL WOJTYLA, POPE JOHN PAUL II
Shores of Silence, Part I

Breathing—the Essence

Just follow the breath.

Learn it.

Taste it.

Feel it.

Surrender to it.

Let the breath be you.

Feel yourself the breath.

Melt.

Fuse.

From the sleeping state

to the waking state.

Let yourself be taken to the gods.

... his soul was in flight. His soul was soaring in an air beyond the world and the body he knew was purified in a breath and delivered of incertitude and made radiant and commingled with the element of the spirit ... His throat ached with a desire to cry aloud, the cry of a hawk or eagle on high, to cry piercingly of his deliverance to the winds. This was the call to life to his soul ...

JAMES JOYCE

Portrait of the Artist as a Young Man

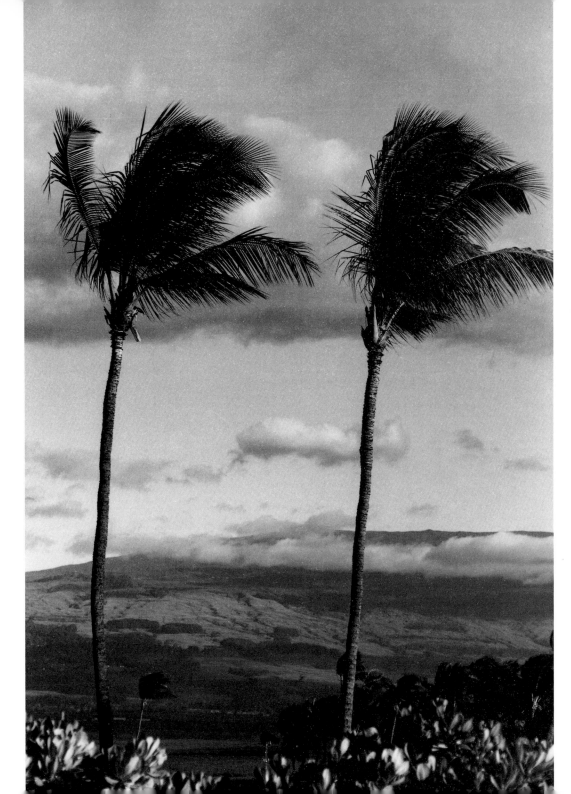

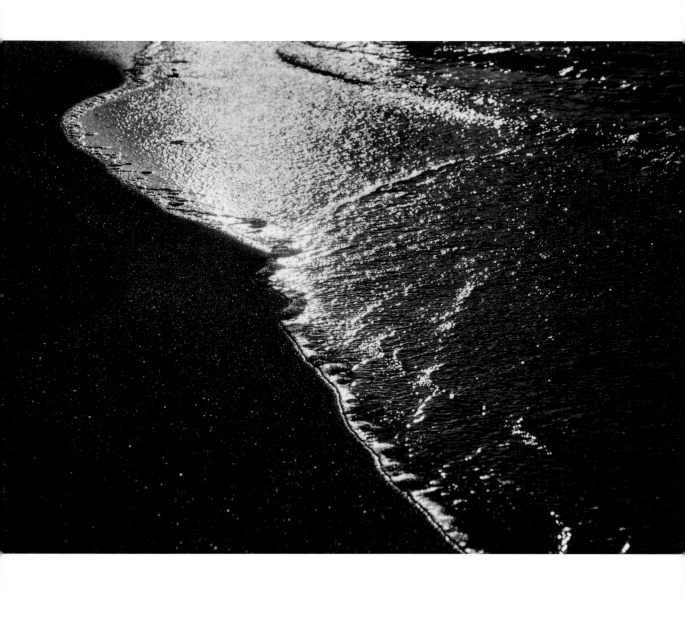

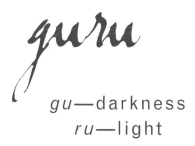

gu—darkness
ru—light

Pranayama is a practice that engages the power of life itself. This is a latent force—capable of destroying the strongest and the weakest. It is only natural that *pranayama* should be taught by a master. Someone who can patiently, with skill and respect for our limitations, bring light to the dark and mysterious.

Such a person is called a *guru*. Whilst we may be taught *asanas* by a teacher, *pranayama* must be supervised by a *guru*.

A *guru* is more than a teacher. A *guru* is someone who lives in the world of energy and spirituality; who guides from experience rather than knowledge; who makes clear the way in which to live our lives.

Chakras

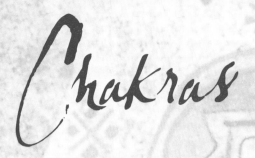

Chakras are inner wheels of energy that are said to control and distribute the flow of *prana* through our bodies.

There are seven major energy centers, located along the spinal column. These vortices of energy may be partially closed, or completely blocked, and need to be opened through practices of purification to function at their full potential.

Each *chakra* represents a state of awareness—a way in which to experience the world. For instance, the second *chakra* is associated with sexuality. For a person living primarily from this *chakra*, everything will be impregnated with this feeling. Sensuality will be of primary importance in this person's life. Similarly, a person residing in the third *chakra*, the center of personal power, will be driven by a competitive edge to conquer and control.

It is only when the *chakras* are evenly balanced that a person settles into a state of harmony.

Pranayama helps to cleanse the toxins that create blockages in the *chakras*. It awakens, releases, and harmonizes.

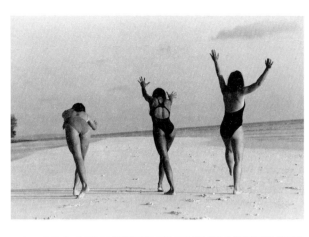

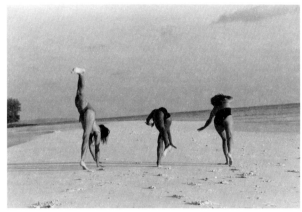

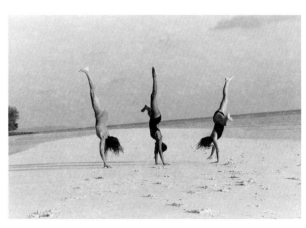

Nadis

Blood runs through the veins. *Prana* runs through the *nadis*.

There are thousands of *nadis* that form a network of energy communication within the skeletal structure. The *susumna, ida,* and *pingala* are the most important.

The *susumna* rises from the base of the spine and runs through the spinal column itself. The *ida* and *pingala* also originate at the base of the spine, but flow on either side of the spine—the *ida* on the left, the *pingala* on the right. These *nadis* are like our main arteries. If they are blocked, the blood of life— *prana*—cannot flow.

Pranayama helps to cleanse the *nadis* so that *prana* can flow clearly and unimpeded through the body. When these *nadis* are alive and rich in free-flowing natural vibrations, we experience life on a high.

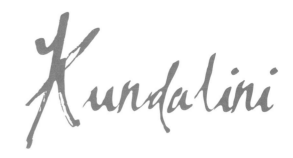

Kundalini

In most people the lower end of the *susumna* is sealed, blocking access to an incredible energy called *kundalini*. The yogis describe this latent power that resides at the base of the spine as a snake coiled three and a half times.

When the impurities are burnt away, the serpent energy is released and begins its ascent of the body. This is a moment of great power. It is accessing a force greater than you.

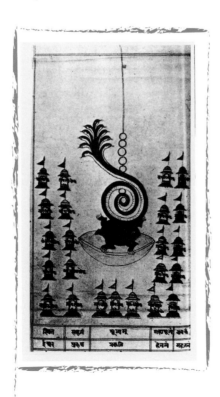

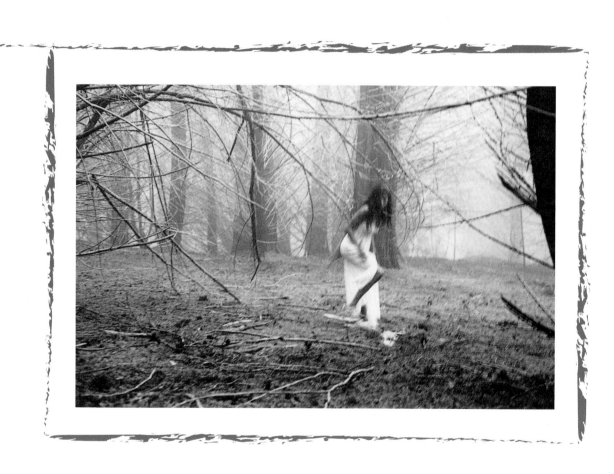

The Breathing

An absolute

patience.

Trees stand

up to their knees in

fog. The fog

slowly flows

uphill.

    White

cobwebs, the grass

leaning where deer

have looked for apples.

The woods

from the brook to where

the top of the hill looks

over the fog, send up

not one bird.

So absolute, it is

no other than

happiness itself, a breathing

too quiet to hear.

DENISE LEVERTOV

The Fourth Stage of the Breath

In and out.

Out and in.

Beyond this flow lies the space within the two.

Retention.

Beyond this lies the fourth state.

Non-breathing.

In this state the breath is so reduced, so shallow, that it becomes a secret.

Undetectable to the outer world.

The mind is still.

The body's own intelligence has taken over.

It feels itself in harmony with the outer world.

The outer and inner become one in their natural state.

There is no mental perception of breath.

There is only allowing and experiencing.

The fourth state only happens in sensitive states of consciousness. According to Patanjali, it unveils the light of truth and tells us that the mind is now fit for practice of *dharana*—focused attention.

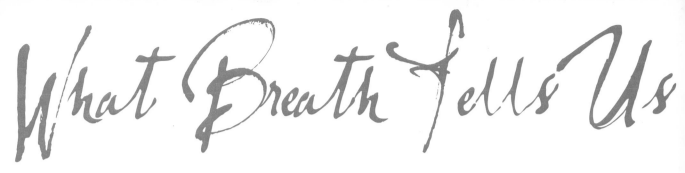

What Breath Tells Us

Start to notice your breath patterns.
When you're in the car and running late.
When you're engaged in a difficult conversation.
When you're anxious. When you're angry.

Notice how your breath morphs, according to your mood, your state of mind, the pace of your day.

Notice when you are irritable how your breath is quick and unsteady.
Then, taking a deep inhale, watch how your mood changes, how the turmoil and tension eases, and the breath becomes quiet and calm.

Breath is your guide. An inner mirror. A narrator.
Always with you, ever-present.

> ... respect for life, truth, and patience are all indispensable factors in the drawing of a quiet breath, in calmness of mind and firmness of will.
>
> YEHUDI MENUHIN

Breath is the outer world coming into one's body. With pulse –
the two always harmonizing – the source of our inward sense of
rhythm. Breath is spirit, "inspiration." Expiration, "voiced,"
makes the signals by which the species connects.
Certain emotions and states occasionally seize the body; one
becomes a whole tube of air vibrating – all voice. In mantra
chanting, the magic utterances, built of seed-syllables such as
OM and AYNG and AH, repeated over and over, fold and furl on
the breath until – when most weary and bored – a new voice
enters, a voice speaks through you clearer and stronger than
what you know of yourself; with a sureness and melody of its
own, singing out the inner song of the self, and of the planet.

GARY SNYDER
Earth House Hold

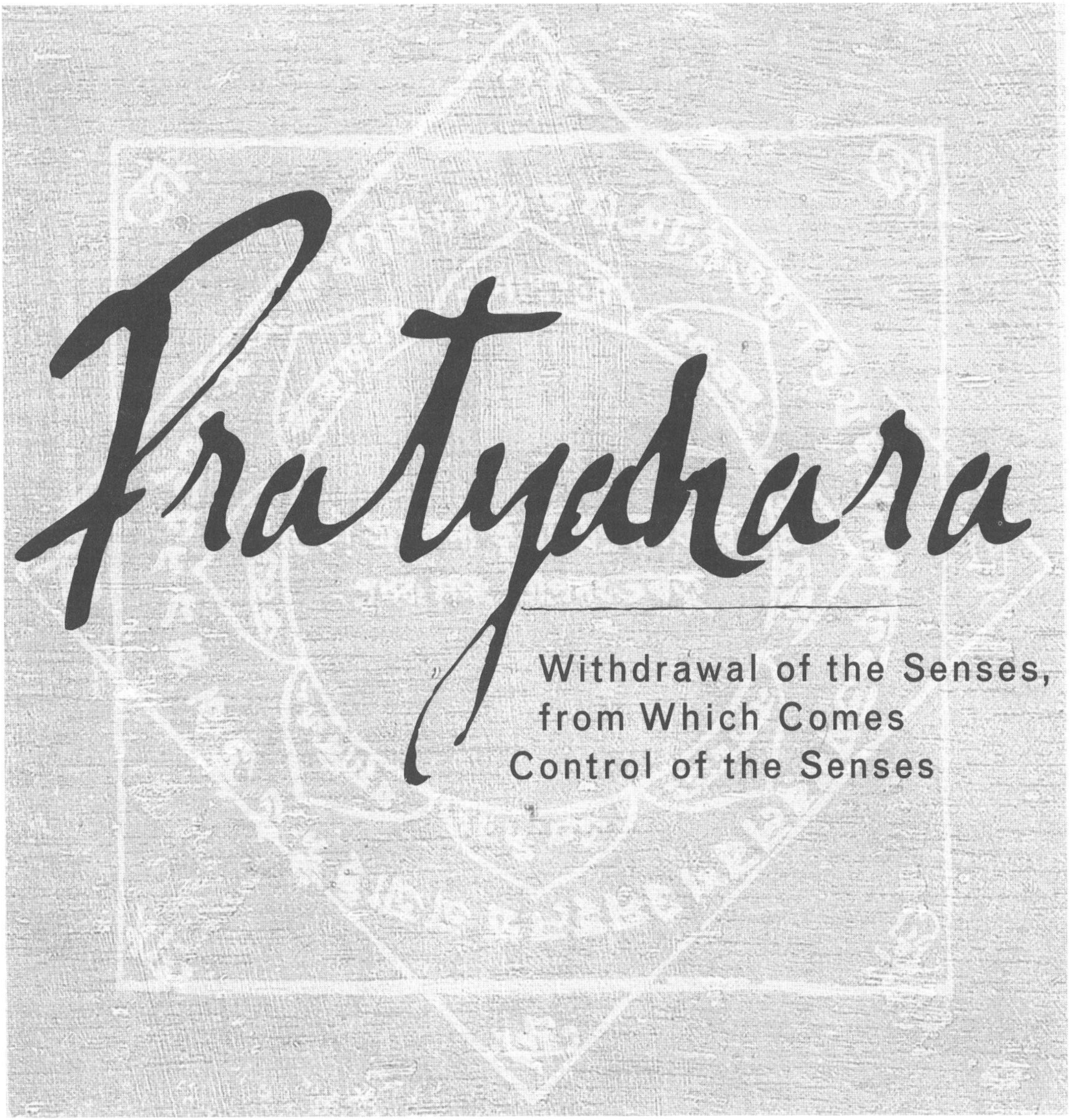

Pratyahara

Withdrawal of the Senses,
from Which Comes
Control of the Senses

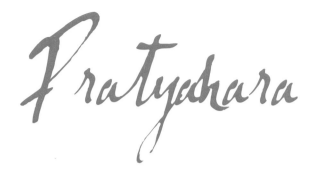

Pratyahara

Pratyahara, the fifth limb of the eightfold path, is concerned with the practice of further internalization and mind control, through the training and withdrawal of the senses. It is the bridge to meditation.

The practice of *asanas* and *pranayama*, *yama* and *niyama*, train the mind and body to turn inwards. *Pratyahara* works directly on furthering this internalization.

Like a charioteer, the person practicing *pratyahara* must bring his senses together—under one rein—moving in one direction, at his command.

The disunited mind is far from wise; how can it meditate? For the unmeditative there is no peace; for the unpeaceful, how can there be happiness? For the mind which yields to the wandering senses carries away his wisdom as a gale carries away a ship on waters.

The Bhagavad Gita (II.66–7)

Train your senses to be obedient.

Regulate your activities to lead you

To the goal. Hold the reins of your mind

As you hold the reins of wild horses.

Svetasvatara Upanishad (II.9)

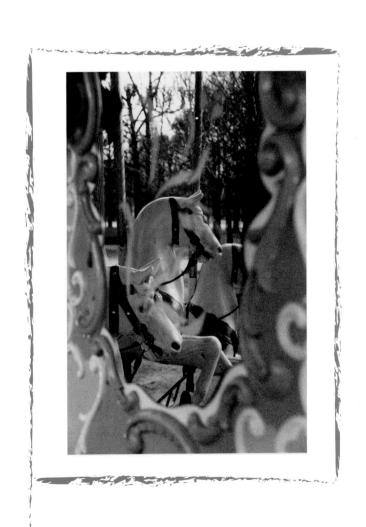

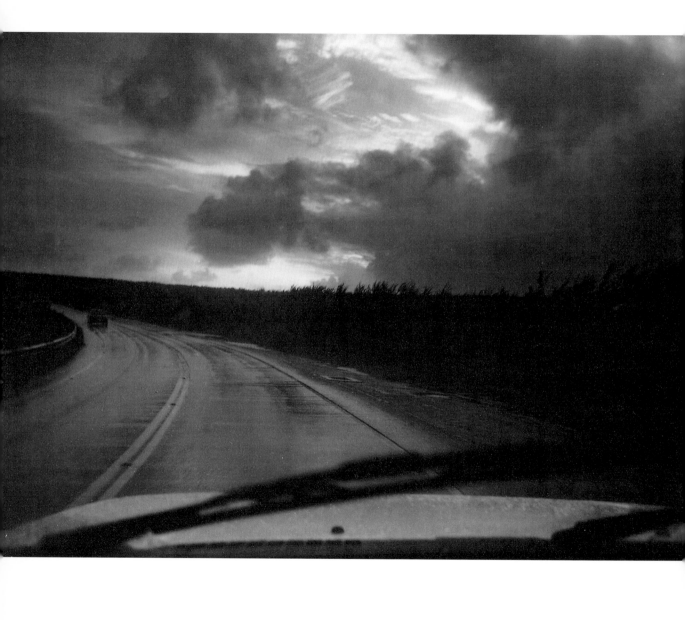

The Self

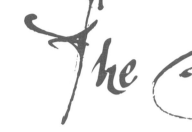

Why withdraw the senses?
What are we looking for?
A meeting with our Self.

What is the Self?

Imagine a glass.
You hold the glass in the ocean.
There is water inside the glass, there is water outside the glass.
The water is the same, but outside the glass it is the Universal Self.
Inside the glass is the Individual Self.

When we are so intensely focused that the sense of separateness disappears,
true Self—*atman*—is experienced. Atman is beyond gender and physicalities.
Atman is beyond time and change.

> Dive
> in the Ocean,
> leave
> and let the sea
> be you.
>
> RUMI

Sense Withdrawal

Withdrawal of the senses does not mean sense negation. On the contrary.
By learning to control the senses you are fine-tuning them. Rather like a
sensitive radio: you are capable of receiving a wide variety of external stimuli but you carefully tune yourself to the frequency of 101 Atman FM. To
the exclusion of all other stations. Until everything else ceases to exist.

This is *pratyahara*.

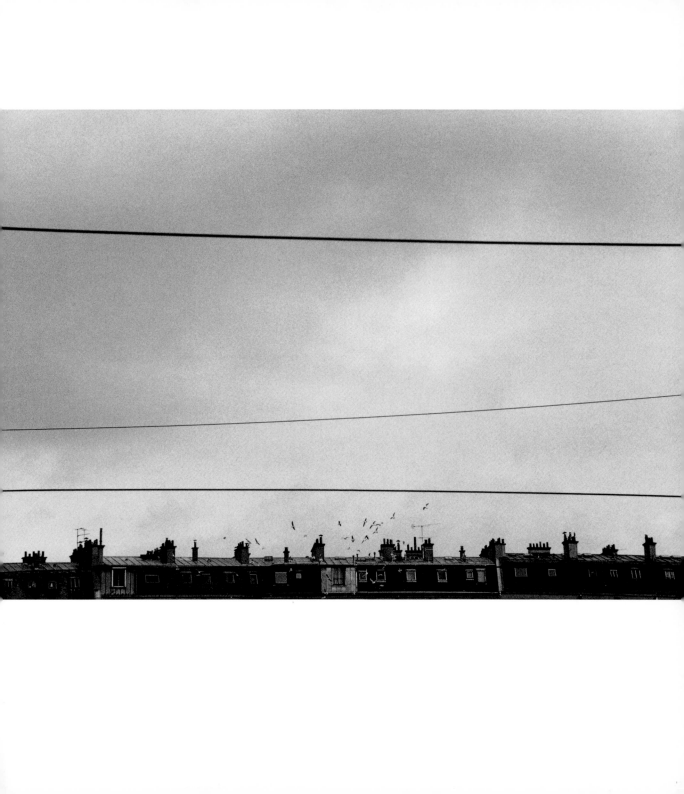

Pratyahara Awakens the Senses

By practicing the withdrawal of the senses we actually explore our senses more deeply than ever before. It is only when trying to focus ourselves in one direction that we realize what an important part the senses play in our day-to-day life.

The taste, the feel, the smell, the noise of things—we are constantly engaged in feeling and reacting to a plethora of sensations. The practice of *pratyahara* brings a new awareness to the senses by acknowledging them fully before attempting to train them. It gives them intensity and subtlety.

It awakens the senses.

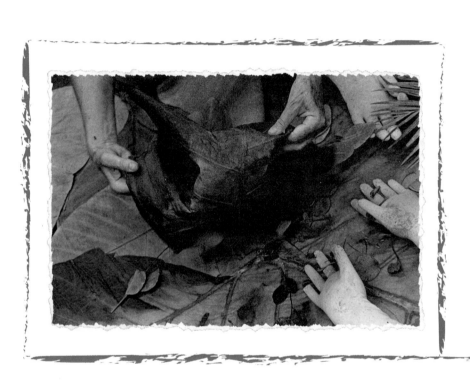

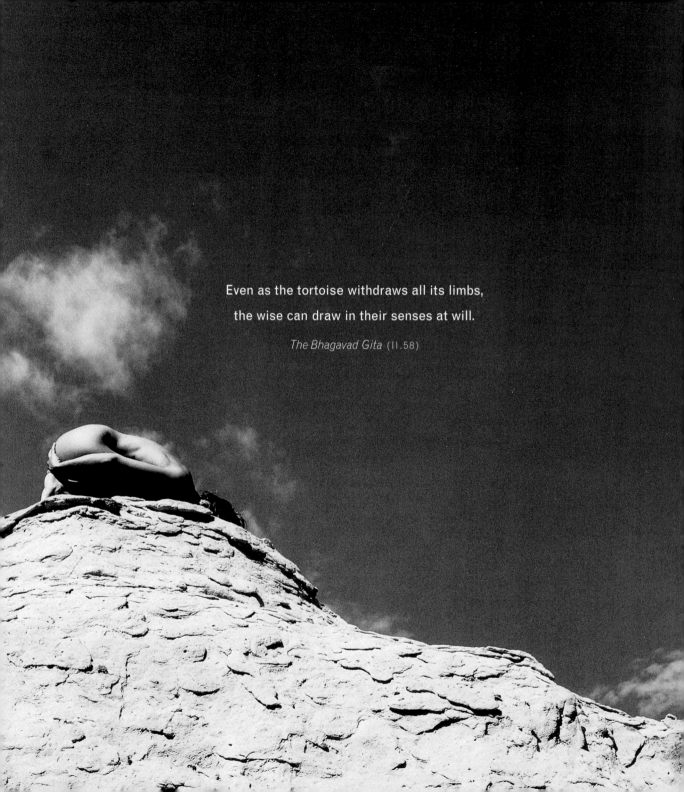

Even as the tortoise withdraws all its limbs,

the wise can draw in their senses at will.

The Bhagavad Gita (II.58)

The World of Pratyahara

Through the practice of *shavasana* and *pranayama* you enter a world of deeper stillness and clarity—a cool inner labyrinth of freshness.

secret
fertile
waiting to be explored

experienced

discovered

Engaging with Awakened Senses

But if I eat an apple, I like to eat with all my senses awake.

Hogging it down like a pig I call the feeding of corpses.

D. H. LAWRENCE
Mystic

Bring your practice of sense withdrawal to each part of your life.

By withdrawing your senses from contact with everything but the object of your attention, you are awakening the potential to discover and swim in the essence of the object itself.

Not practicing sense withdrawal, or sense awakening, is like being half-asleep. You are missing the simple subtleties of your existence.

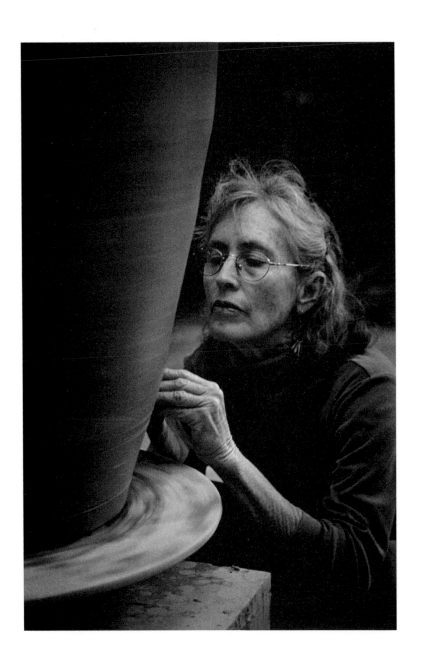

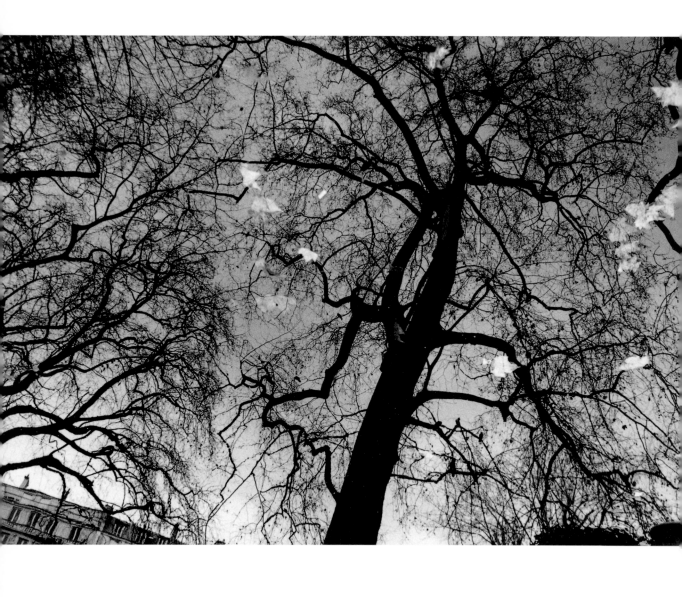

Every pore finds peace, as you slip from the practice of *pratyahara* to a state of focused awareness.

Slipping through the hurdles of galaxy trash that float through your mind and senses, you find perfect neutrality.

discovering the secret that holds the stars apart

But when one loves amidst the world of sense, free from attachment and aversion alike, such a person attains serenity. And from serenity results cessation of all his sufferings. For in a person with a serene mind, wisdom soon becomes firmly set.

The Bhagavad Gita (II.64–5)

Pratyahara is not about doing, feeling, and achieving many things. It is about deepening the experience and knowledge of one small particular thing. A blade of grass, the smell of your child, the sound of one piece by Mozart, your breath, your inner body.

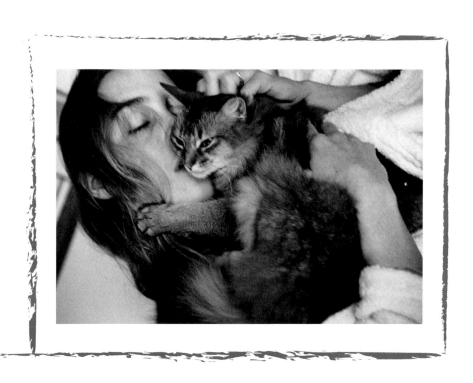

Practicing Pratyahara

There are many ways to practice *pratyahara*.

Some people like to use a specific yoga posture such as *shavasana*, some use hand gestures (known as *mudras*), and some people cover their eyes and ears to focus in on their inner world.

If you experiment too much with different ideas you will find that your senses are dispersed, so it is better to find one method that works for you and stick to it. Experiment, then choose your prop, and practice regularly within these boundaries.

It is like practicing an *asana* pose over and over again. Although the structure of the pose remains the same, your experience of the pose deepens and deepens.

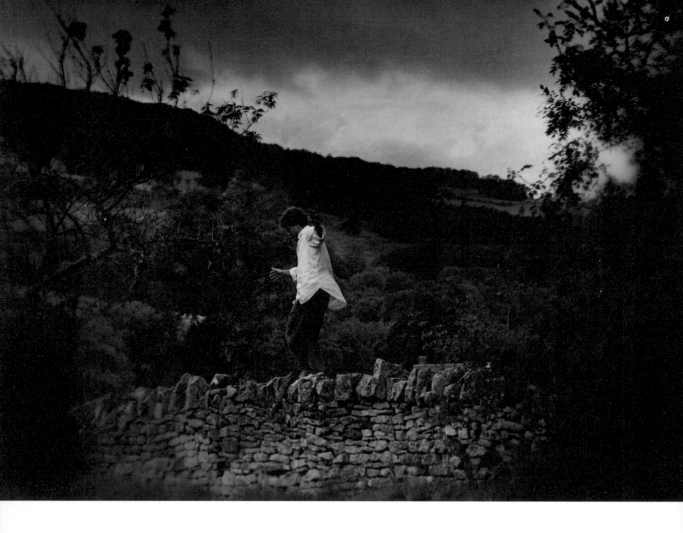

The world of the senses gives rise to heat and cold, pleasure and pain.

They come and they go and do not last. Bear them patiently.

For a person unmoved by these changes, for whom sorrow and

happiness are the same is truly wise, and fit for immortality.

The Bhagavad Gita (II:14–15)

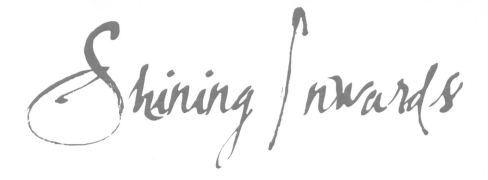

Shining Inwards

We never really encounter the world. What we experience is our own nervous system reacting to the world.

Physics teaches us that everything is energy and that at its deepest level all things are interconnected. We see things as separate because of the limitation of our senses. This sense of separateness is an illusion.

The Self is beyond the senses. It stands apart—free and knowing. To experience the Self—this infinite reality beneath the world of the senses—our consciousness needs to shine inwards away from external stimuli.

This is the slow journey away from the duality of the senses and the mind, to unity and stillness. To a soul that has poise.

The River Metaphor

Pratyahara—Withdrawal of the senses
Dharana—Focused attention
Dhyana—Meditation
Samadhi—Self-realization

Pratyahara, dharana, dhyana and *samadhi* can be compared to
a boat journey on a river.

When you set out on the boat, you leave behind the land,
the trees, the bustle of community.
Your senses begin to merge with the experience of the river.
This is *pratyahara*.

As the journey progresses, you become more and more detached from
what you left behind. And more and more immersed in the rhythm
of the water. You are floating, melting, gurgling—you feel the river in
your veins, your flesh, in the taste on your tongue.
This is *dharana*—mental absorption.

Dhyana, a state of meditation, naturally follows.

In this state you and the river are one. The boat disappears.

You are the river—dancing through light, over reeds, across land.

Then, when the river finally flows into the sea,

your I-ness completely disappears.

This is *samadhi*.

The dissolution of dichotomies.

The boat, your Self, the river, the sea.

All are one.

Dharana

Focused Attention

Yoga is restraint of the mind stuff.

PATANJALI

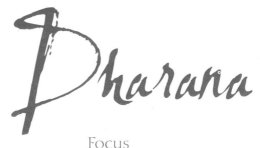

Dharana

Focus
Attention
Concentration
Connection

Dharana, the sixth limb of yoga, is the state of mental focus that precedes meditative absorption.

Imagine a beautiful tree.

You sit down. You admire.

You engage.

So intently that eventually you lose all sense of things unrelated to that tree.

You forget about your headache, the cars behind you, the problems at work, your fatigue …

All of your senses are serving the mind.

You are intently focused.

Everything in you connects to the tree.

Every atom is directed towards the tree.

Flowing.

Like a river.

You dissolve, until there is fusion.

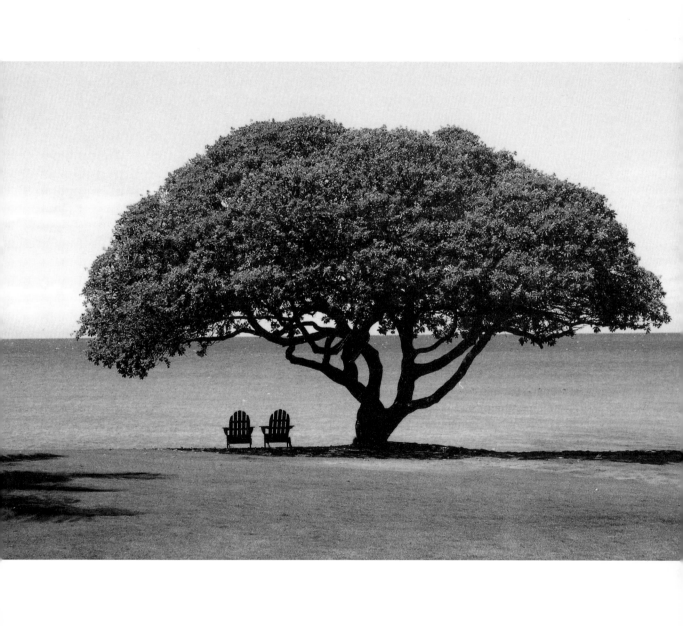

The Birds Have Vanished

The birds have vanished into the sky,
And how the last cloud drains away.

We sit together, the mountain and me,
Until only the mountain remains.

LI PO

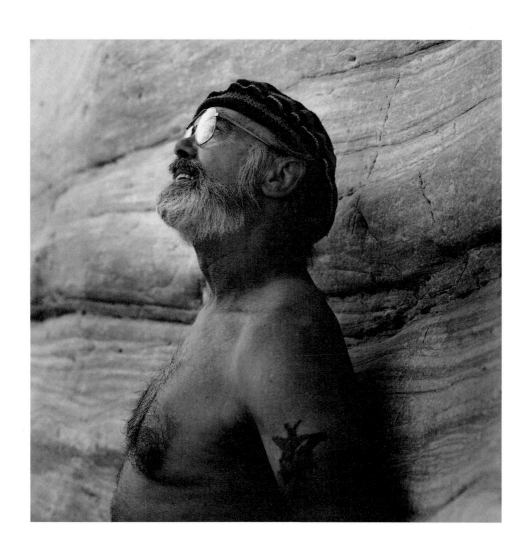

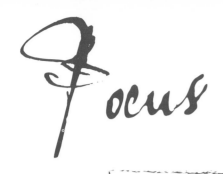

Focus

> ## As a lamp in a sheltered spot does not flicker.
>
> *The Bhagavad Gita*

Imagine yourself in a dark basement, flashlight in hand, looking for an old photo album. The batteries in your light are old and the light is weak and vapid. You can only make out shadows and shapes.

But once you change the batteries your flashlight emits a powerful directional beam. You find what you are looking for easily. The light picks it out from the clutter and lights it up intensely.

Dharana is part of this process—the transformation from dispersedness to one-pointedness.

By shining the light of awareness where there was murkiness and darkness before, you start to see what is inside and around you.

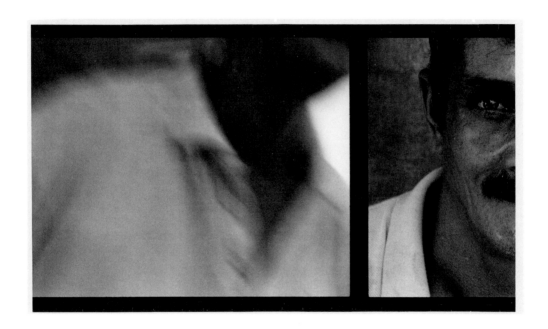

Concentration is to bind consciousness to a single spot.

PATANJALI

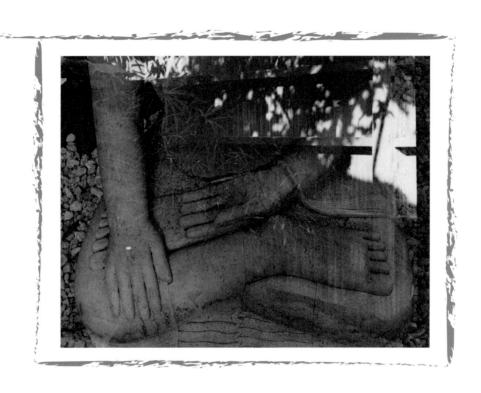

To a mind that's still the whole universe surrenders.

LAO-TZU

Tao-Te-Ching

Practicing Focused Attention

When practicing *dharana*, the object of attention can be anything so long as it helps you to focus. Anything on which the gaze or attention can be fixed—a stone, an apple, a cup, a coin, a candle, the body, the breath. What is important is that the object of attention is pleasant to focus on. Then the practice is simply to fix the mind on the object and hold the attention there.

Pick a quiet time.

Sit comfortably, letting yourself be at ease and yet alert.

Now direct your consciousness to a single point, to the object of attention.

Hold your mind there, unwavering, absolutely concentrated.

Let go of all concepts, associations, and reflections—all connections that might limit your perception of it.

Open yourself to the object with the wonder and freshness of a young child.

Let it fill your entire mind.

Make every moment an act of engagement.

Wherever you are going. Whatever you are doing.

Bring your entire being to the moment.

Invest one hundred percent awareness into the mundane.

Use each and every opportunity as an inspiration to practice focused attention.

Washing the dishes to wash the dishes

At first glance that might seem a little silly: why put so much stress on a simple thing? But that's precisely the point. The fact that I am standing there washing the bowls is a wondrous reality. I'm being completely myself, following my breath, conscious of my presence, and conscious of my thoughts and actions. There's no way I can be tossed around mindlessly like a bottle slapped here and there on the waves.

THICH NHAT HANH

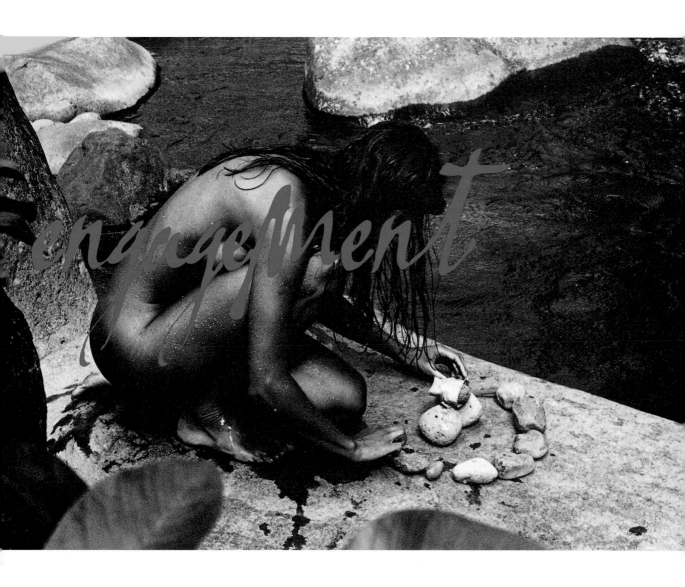

In time, with regular practice of *dharana*, the object on which you focus will become more vivid and luminous. In other words, your perception of that object, filtered through your senses and emotions, will change. The true nature of the object, irrespective of your mind, will begin to be known. Its pure essence revealed.

These subtle levels of consciousness are the gift of the practice of *dharana*.

The moon's the same old moon,
The flowers exactly as they were,
Yet I've become the thingness
of all the things I see!

BUNAN

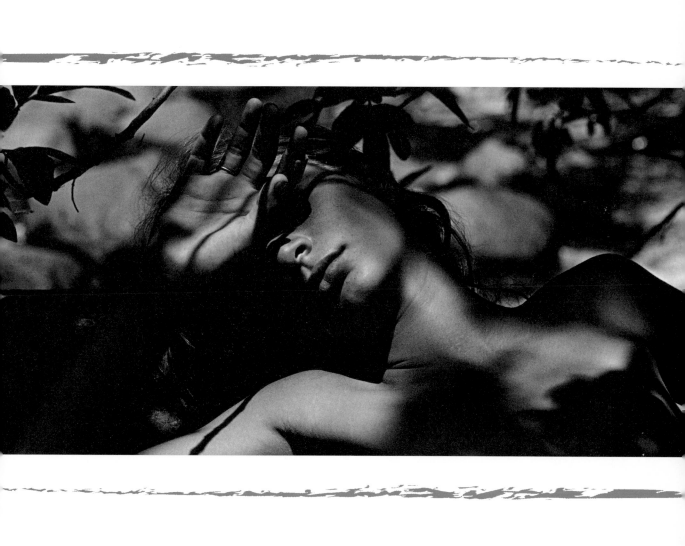

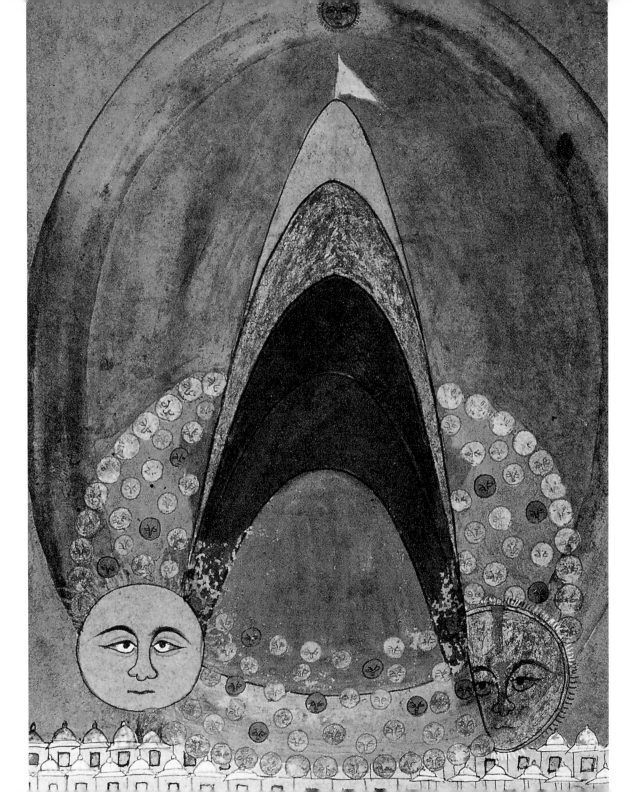

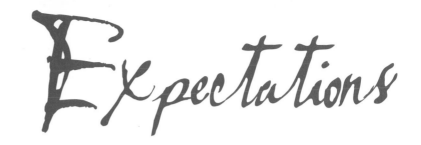

Expectations

Don't let the goals of your practice get in the way. As you practice focused awareness, you will find that your mind starts to want or expect things to happen. I should be happier! I should be more peaceful! I should be less chaotic in my life!

Although a still and relaxed state may result from mindfulness, the true purpose is to directly experience things as they are, as they come and go. If you're sitting with expectations then you are not in contact with the present moment, which contains the whole of life. The practice of focused attention strengthens the muscle of awareness as a muscle in your body might be strengthened. Eventually, when the muscle is strong and constant, an inner softness—the state of *being* in meditation—can flow through.

Midnight. No waves

no wind, the empty boat

is flooded with moonlight.

DOGEN

We must continue to open in the face of tremendous opposition. No one is
encouraging us to open and still we must peel away the layers of the heart.

CHÖGYAM TRUNGPA RINPOCHE

Focused attention is the beginning of meditation. When we practice we are
offering our willingness to be here for whatever life offers. This is neither
supported nor encouraged by the exterior hectic world or the interior
muddle of your mind.

Every message is to switch off.

Come this way. Come that way.

Try this. Try that.

It is a very difficult thing to stay on your seat and just be there for
whatever turns up.

We have to learn to sit and be open to whatever arrives.

Creativity and Dharana

Observe the immersion of an artist, such as a painter, a photographer, or a musician.

For the painter, there is nothing but the object being painted and the emotional reinterpretation of this thing. For the photographer, all that exists is the urge to capture the feeling, the mood, the essence of the scene. For the musician, each note becomes a study and reflection of Self—an outpouring of soul.

The very nature of being an artist demands that you attempt to connect with intensity each time you engage in your art. It requires you to let go of all other realities, to immerse yourself in the state of attention needed to truly fuse, feel, understand, and eventually express.

Deep creative engagement is total focused absorption. *Dharana*.

The flowering of *pratyahara* and *dharana* is *dhyana*. Meditation.
And *dhyana* then leads us to the nectar of yoga—*samadhi*—self-realization.

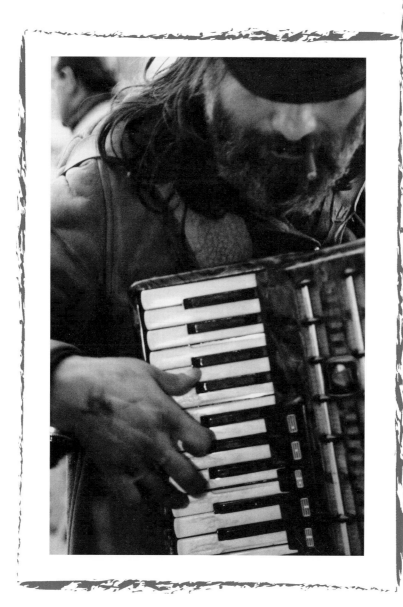

If you want to understand the beauty of a bird, a fly, or a leaf, or a person with all his complexities, you have to give your whole attention, which is awareness ... Such awareness is like living with a snake in the room; you watch its every movement, you are very, very sensitive to the slightest sound it makes. Such a state of attention is total energy; in such awareness the totality of yourself is revealed in an instant.

J. KRISHNAMURTI

Dhyana

Meditation

At the still point of the turning world
... at the still point there the dance is.

T. S. ELIOT

What is Meditation?

Stopping and looking deeply into the nature of what is there.

A direct experience, rather than an interpretation

of direct experience.

A stilling of the mind.

Meditation is a practice that denies nothing.

It is living with the doors and windows open.

The wind of the world blows though, commingling with the breath of Self.

Letting go and allowing that wind to carry you.

The answer my friend is blowing in the wind ...

BOB DYLAN

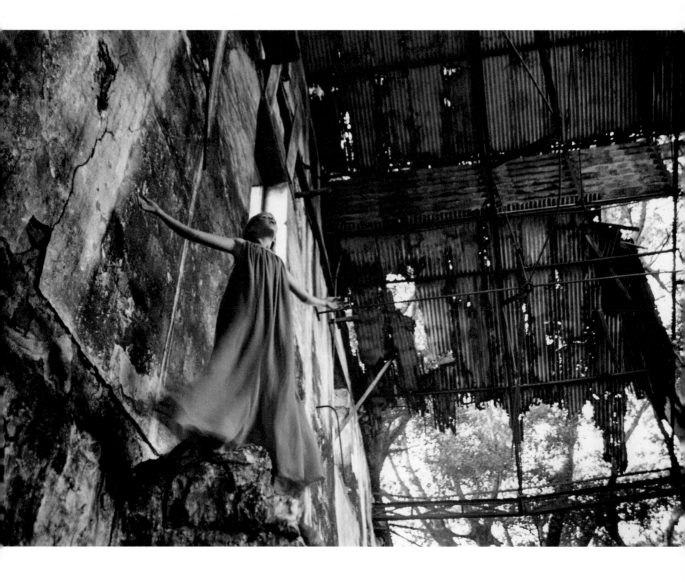

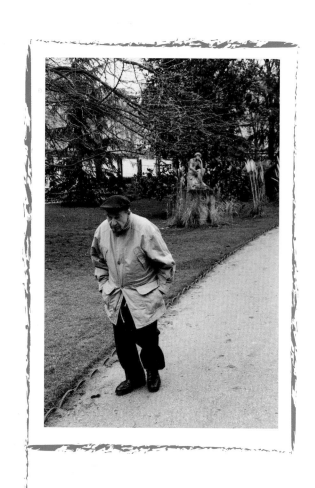

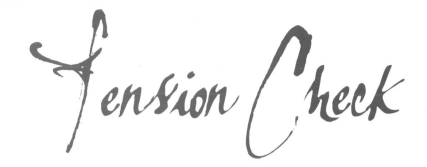

Tension Check

Notice how your body feels right now. Are your shoulders a little hunched, is your jaw tight and clenched, or relaxed? Notice what you are thinking about, what your concerns and preoccupations are in this moment. What is the flavor of your thoughts? And your contact with the outside world: is there movement in the air, which touches your skin? Notice the feel of your body against a chair or cushion or the floor. Be in direct experience.

With *dhyana*, the seventh limb of the eightfold path, we begin to look deeply and develop insight into the nature of things.

A little boy asked his mother, "Mummy, what is meditation?"

The mother sat down and explained that meditation is when you focus very intently on one thing, for a long time, until eventually the essence of the thing reveals itself. And then you see it for what it really is.

The little boy went away and thought about it.

A few days later he came to his mother and said, "Mummy, can we meditate on a bicycle?"

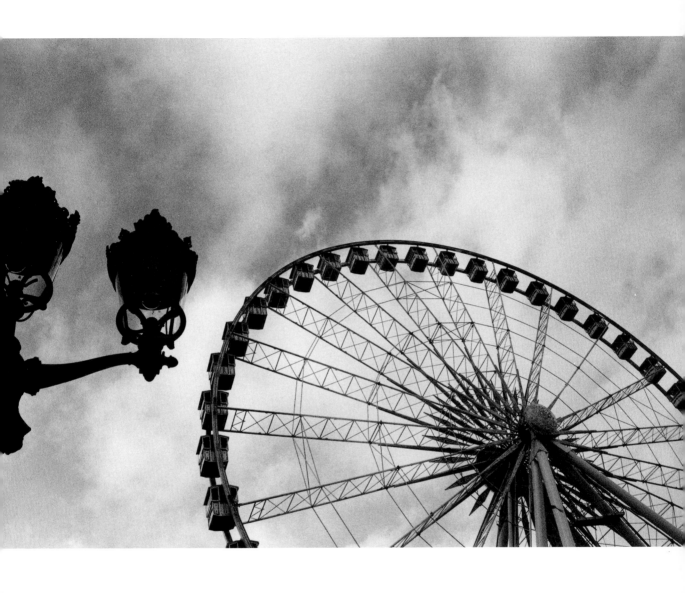

Two Types of Meditation

There are two approaches to meditation: meditation with a focus, and objectless awareness.

Focused meditation is easier. Attention is narrowed to a specific focus, which helps to keep you anchored in the present moment. There is a variety of ways to do this, such as following the movement of the breath, repeating a sacred phrase or mantra, or through an action like eating, walking or washing dishes. Once you have chosen a focus, stick to it with commitment and steadiness, bringing yourself back to the practice again and again each time your mind deviates.

Objectless awareness is pure mindfulness. Welcoming whatever enters the field of your consciousness. Stories, temptations, sounds, physical sensations. Your only job is to stay where you are and observe what comes and goes.

Both approaches require stamina. This stamina is strengthened through committed practice.

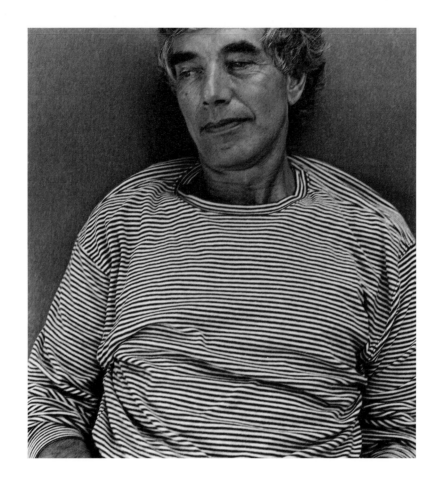

What is Yoga?

A resting point.

For myself.

For all people that I come in contact with.

ARTIST

The gentle practice

When you begin to meditate, you will notice how much is going on in your mind. It pulls you here and there, back and forth, over and over again.

The untrained mind is restless and repetitive by nature. It doesn't care about your need for peace and stillness. It just goes ahead and invents its novels, presents its fantasies, and unravels its to-do lists.

Trying to bring the mind under control is like trying to tame the wind. So while meditating it is a challenge to stay present with all that flows through your consciousness. Even with the best intentions you will get caught in the concerns, preoccupations and stories that the mind naturally creates.

Be easy on yourself. Remember, the practice is to gently keep bringing your attention back to the present moment, no matter how many times your mind wanders. Each time simply return.

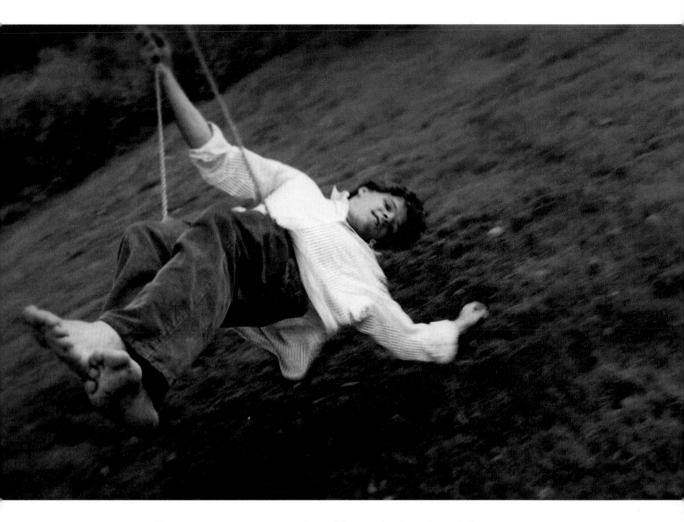

The present moment is where life can be found, and if you

don't arrive there, you miss your appointment with life.

THICH NHAT HANH

Cultivating Attitudes of the Heart

In both Buddhism and Hinduism there is a 2,500-year-old practice where the four noblest qualities of mind are radiated into the universe for the benefit of all living creatures.

This special meditation exercise cultivates friendliness, compassion, joy, and peace of mind. It is a practice that develops a spacious heart.

may all beings be happy
may all beings be filled with joy
may all beings be free from suffering
may all beings know peace

Sit comfortably in a quiet place. Bring a soft attention to your breathing. Begin by repeating over and over again these or similar phrases. Reflect on the benefits of these qualities. Imagine the center of your heart opening, and radiating a vast and limitless outpouring of love and tenderness to yourself and all beings.

This meditation has not been around for thousands of years for nothing. It is powerful. It can transform.

Heart

My heart

Is broken

Open.

RICK FIELDS

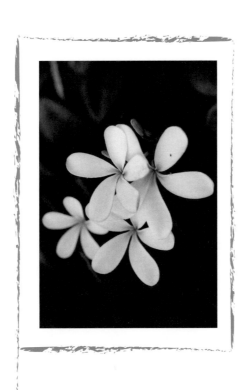

Siddhis

As the yogi gains subtlety through mastery of the mind and senses, paranormal abilities, such as supernatural hearing and sight, can be experienced. These are known as *siddhis*—special gifts.

Unfortunately, these gifts also come with a dark side—they are sometimes so overwhelming that the weaker person will find it impossible to resist their temptation. This person will lose sight of *moksha*—true and total freedom. So, whilst *siddhis* are extraordinary, they are also yogic tests of character in themselves.

We must remember that such powers are not the aim of yoga. They may be a by-product of the yogic practice, but they should never be considered goals in themselves.

It is not always understood that meditation, as the keystone of any yogic discipline, is a highly potent instrument which, like nuclear power, can be put to constructive or destructive use.

GEORG FEUERSTEIN

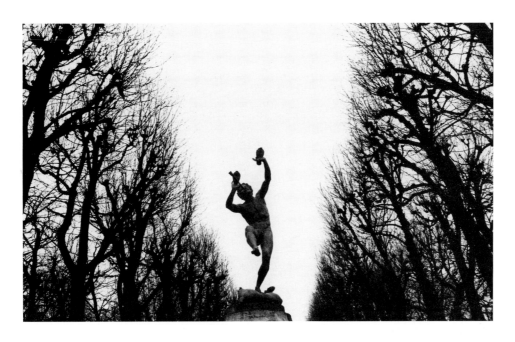

You'll get mixed up, of course,

as you already know.

You'll get mixed up

with many strange birds as you go.

So be sure when you step.

Step with care and great tact

and remember that Life's a Great Balancing Act.

Just never forget to be dexterous and deft.

And *never* mix your right foot with your left.

DR SEUSS

Oh, the Places You'll Go

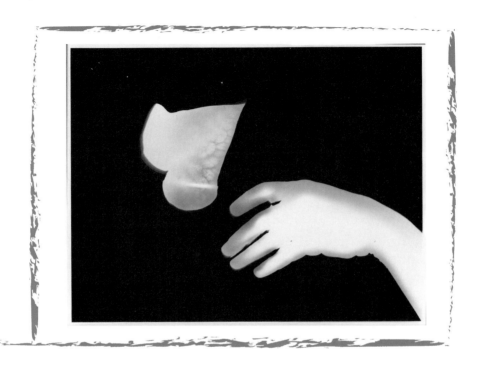

When I speak of love I am not speaking of some
sentimental and weak response, I am speaking of that
force which all great religions have seen as the supreme
unifying principle of life. Love is somehow the key that
unlocks the door which leads to ultimate reality.

MARTIN LUTHER KING, JR.

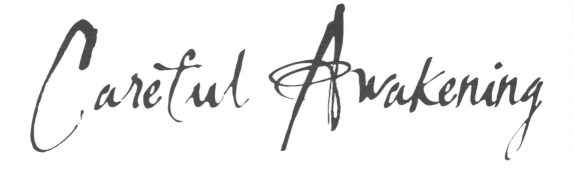

Careful Awakening

As we awaken, we must maintain humility and respect. Partial awakening of consciousness can be dangerous. It can make us think more of ourselves than we should.

Much like an average driver who decides to take a Ferrari out for a spin. Not thoroughly grounded in the subtleties of such a high powered machine, they could create an accident at any moment.

Keep the ego in check. Drive the Renault.

As our body, heart, mind, and spirit open, each new layer we encounter reveals both greater freedom and compassion and deeper and more subtle layers of underlying delusion.

JACK KORNFIELD

Meditation is a state in which we find ourselves after much practice of inwardness and awareness.
It is a gift.
It is a prelude to *samadhi*.

Meditation is the highest form of prayer, and what is prayer but the expansion of your Self into living cosmos?

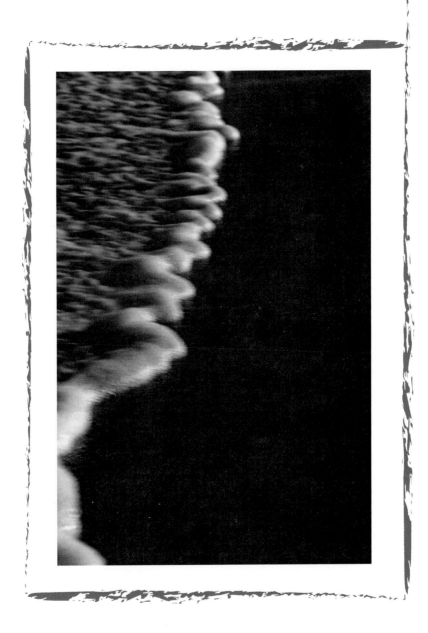

Siddhartha listened. He was now listening intently, completely absorbed, quite empty, taking in everything. He felt that he had now completely learned the art of listening. He had often heard all this before, all these numerous voices in the river, but today they sounded different. He could no longer distinguish the different voices – the merry voice from the weeping voice, the childish voice from the manly voice. They all belonged to each other: the lament of those who yearn, the laughter of the wise, the cry of indignation and the groan of the dying. They were all interwoven and interlocked, entwined in a thousand ways. And all the voices, all the goals, all the yearnings, all the sorrows, all the pleasures, all the good and evil, all of them together was the world. All of them together was the stream of events, the music of life. When Siddhartha listened attentively to this river, to this song of a thousand voices; when he did not listen to the sorrow or the laughter, when he did not bind his soul to any one particular voice and absorb it in his Self, but heard them all, the whole, the unity; then the great song of a thousand voices consisted of one word: Om – perfection.

HERMAN HESSE
Siddhartha

Samadhi

Enlightenment. Self-realization

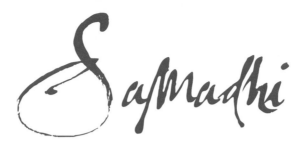

Self-realization

Samadhi is the merging of the perceiver with the perceived, the subject with the object, the grasper with the grasped.

It is not a practice. It is the conclusion to our practice. It is the shift from the conscious Self to the transcendental Self. It is coming home. It is when the Self abides in its own essence.

Samadhi is the last part of Patanjali's eightfold path. It is the final gift of yoga.

It is seeing the soul face to face, an absolute indivisible state of existence in which all differences between body, mind and soul are dissolved.

B. K. S. IYENGAR

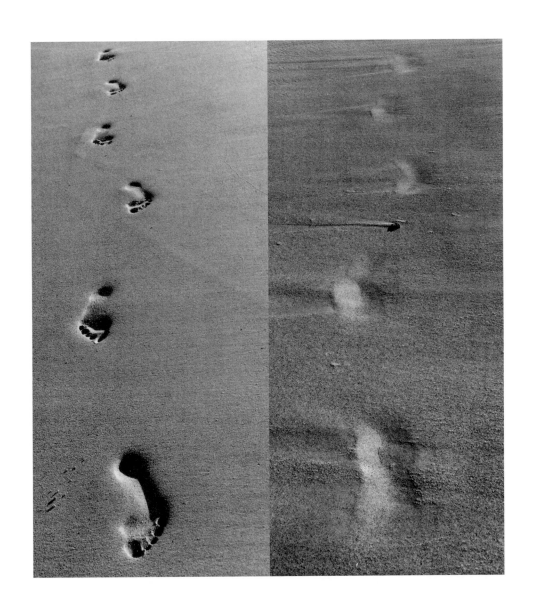

Let go of the idea "I exist"

IKKUY

ECSTASY

Joy triggered from outside
From a source external and separate

ENSTASY

Joy emerging from within
Dwelling in our true essence
Experiencing the transcendental Self

Samadhi

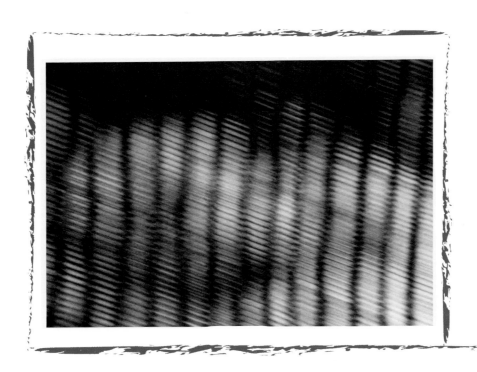

It was but yesterday I thought

    myself a fragment

Quivering without rhythm in the sphere

    of life.

Now I know that I am the sphere

    and all life in

Rhythmic fragments moves within me.

KAHLIL GIBRAN

The yogis believe that the inherent nature of this world is one of sorrow.

Man's most basic desire is to carve a foothold in the ever-changing chaos of life; to create a platform of stability in a fluid, fluctuating world. And man discovers time and time again that nothing ever remains the same. Everything moves, everything changes. Even the experience of joy is tinged with sorrow. The sorrow of wanting more of that joy. Of wanting to live in the joy and being unable to.

Nevertheless we can transcend this situation with much hard work, practice, and dispassion. We can live beyond it. We can reside in the essence of ourselves.

This is *samadhi*. The underlying aim of yoga.

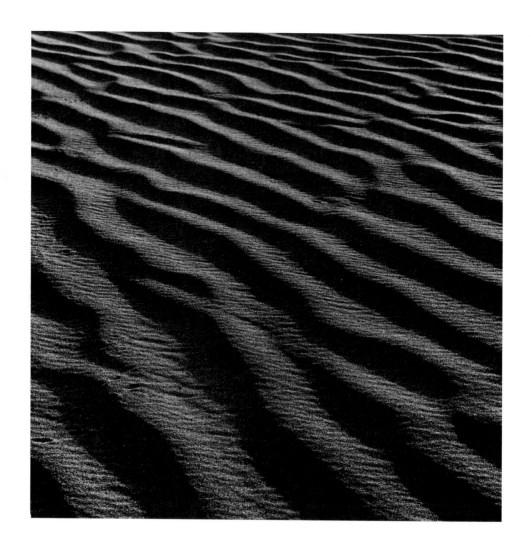

The temple bell stops

But the sound keeps coming

Out of the flowers

BASHO

The Stages of Samadhi

Rare is the awakening to full enlightenment. *Samadhi* is generally experienced in stages—moments of awakening which come and go. Artists and mystics throughout time have described these moments in different ways. Allen Ginsberg wrote this about his first glimpse of intimate awareness:

... Everyday light seemed like sunlight in eternity ... I had the impression of the entire universe as poetry filled with light and intelligence and communication and signals ...

The German medieval mystic Hildegarde experienced it like this:

... The light I perceive ... is much brighter than the cloud which bears the sun ... While I am enjoying the spectacle of this light, all sadness and sorrow vanish from my memory.

Each person experiences it differently yet the same. Joy, love, bliss, understanding, freedom, light. These moments of expanding consciousness that transform us are the precursors to *samadhi*.

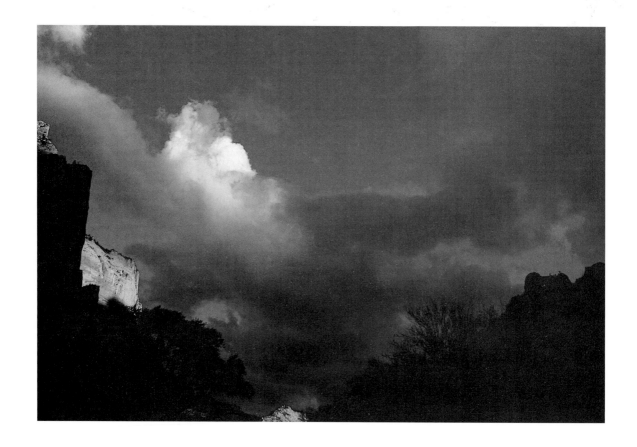

The final stage of *samadhi* is a complete union of subject and object. The seer perceives everything through the superconscious. The mind is dropped. There is total disintegration of past programming. Everything is experienced directly through the Self, in the Self, and of the Self. The seer abides completely in his own essence. The world. The cosmos. God.

The "kingdom of God" isn't
something that one waits for; it has
no yesterday and no tomorrow, it
doesn't come in a thousand years—
it is an experience that takes place
inside the heart; it is everywhere,
it is nowhere.

FRIEDRICH NIETZSCHE

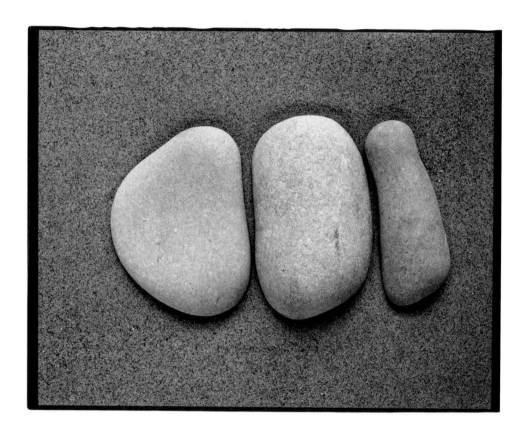

Sound is a vibration, which as modern science tells us, is at the source of all

creation. God is beyond vibration, but vibration, being the subtlest form

of His creation, is the nearest we can get to Him in the physical world.

So we take it as His symbol.

B. K. S. IYENGAR

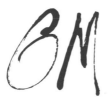

AUM

Om. Sacred symbol.
Sound of the universe. Creation and the Creator.
Samadhi—bliss

Though indivisible it has three sounds. A, U, M.

AAAAAAAAUUUUUUUUMMMMMMMMM

But it is the symbol of OM that represents total transcendence.

This symbol is the sound of liberation.
It stands for humanity's realization that divinity is in the Self.

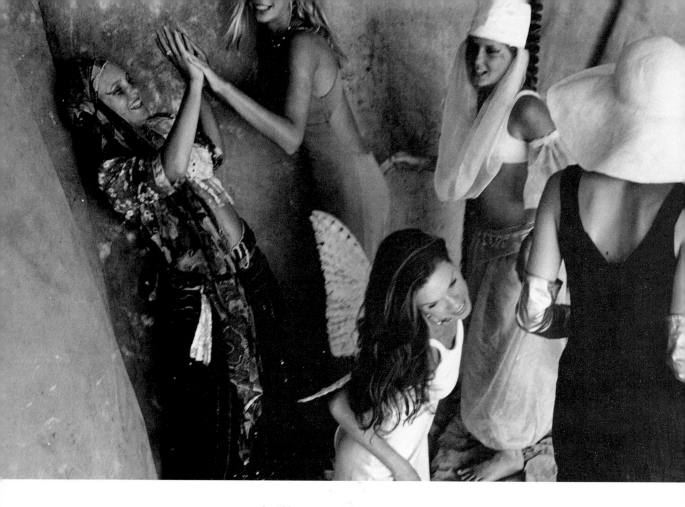

In "Not-two" nothing is separate

and nothing in the world is excluded.

In it there is no gain or loss,

no here, no there,

the tiny is as large as the vast,

the vast as small as the tiny.

In it there is no yesterday, no today, no tomorrow.

SENG TS'AN

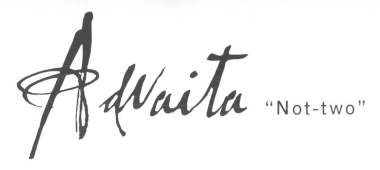 **Advaita** "Not-two"

With *samadhi* every trace of separateness disappears. Duality disappears.
Resting in the knowledge that all things are interconnected. The unity of life.

If you are a poet, you will see clearly that there is a cloud floating in this sheet of paper.
Without a cloud, there will be no rain; without rain, the trees cannot grow; and
without trees, we cannot make paper. The cloud is essential for the paper to exist ...
If we look into this sheet of paper even more deeply, we can see the sunshine
in it. Without sunshine the forest cannot grow. In fact nothing can grow without
sunshine. And so we know that the sunshine is also in this piece of paper. And we
see wheat. We know that the logger cannot exist without his daily bread, and
therefore the wheat that became his bread is also in this sheet of paper. The
logger's mother and father are in it too. When we look in this way, we see that
without all of these things, this sheet of paper cannot exist.
Looking even more deeply we see ourselves in this sheet of paper too. This is not
difficult to see, because when we look at a sheet of paper, it is part of our
perception. Your mind is in here and mine is also. So we can say that everything
is in here with this sheet of paper. We cannot point out one thing that is not
here—time, space, the earth, the rain, the minerals in the soil, the sunshine,
the cloud, the river, the heat. Everything co-exists with this sheet of paper ...
As thin as this piece of paper is, it contains everything in the universe.

THICH NHAT HANH

195

No man is an Island, entire of itself;

Every man is a piece of a continent, a part of the main;

If a clod be washed away by the sea,

Europe is the less, as well as if a promontory were,

As well as if a manor of thy friends or of thine own were;

Any man's death diminishes me, because I am involved in mankind;

And therefore, never send to know for whom the bell tolls,

It tolls for thee.

JOHN DONNE
Meditation XVII

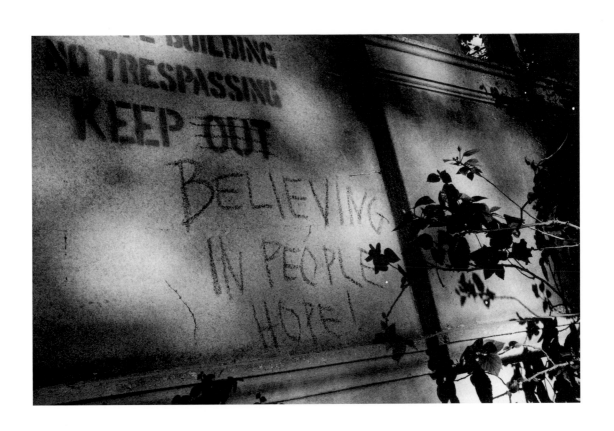

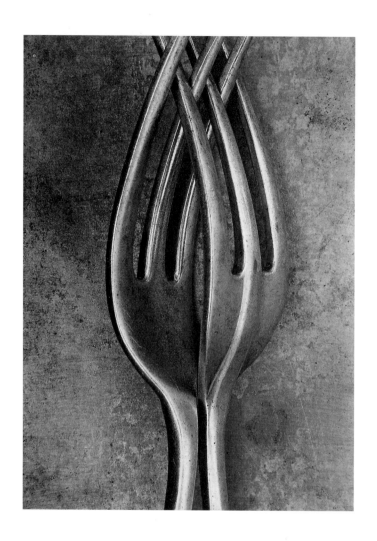

What is Yoga?

Isn't it that thing you do when you all hold hands?

BANKER

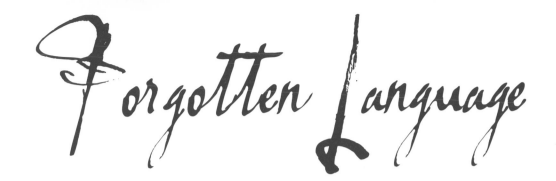

Forgotten Language

Once I spoke the language of flowers,

Once I understood each word the caterpillar said,

Once I smiled in secret at the gossip of starlings,

And shared a conversation with a housefly

in my bed.

Once I heard and answered all the questions

of the crickets,

And joined the crying of each falling dying

flake of snow,

Once I spoke the language of the flowers ...

How did it go?

How did it go?

SHEL SILVERSTEIN
Where the Sidewalk Ends

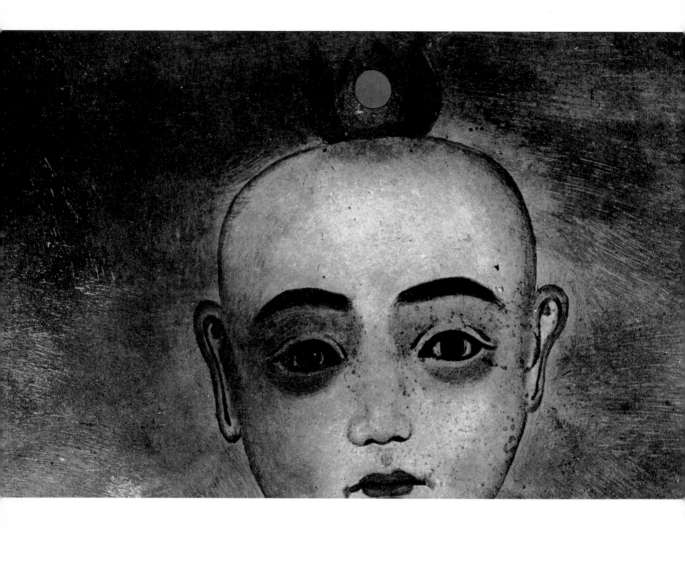

When the mind fluctuations have dwindled, consciousness becomes like a transparent jewel; residing in the pure essence of itself.

PATANJALI

The love of God, unutterable and perfect,

flows into a pure soul the way that light

moves into a transparent object.

The more love that it finds, the more it gives itself;

so that, as we grow clear and open,

the more complete the joy of loving is.

DANTE

The Divine Comedy

seeker of truth

follow no path
all paths lead where

truth is here

e. e. cummings

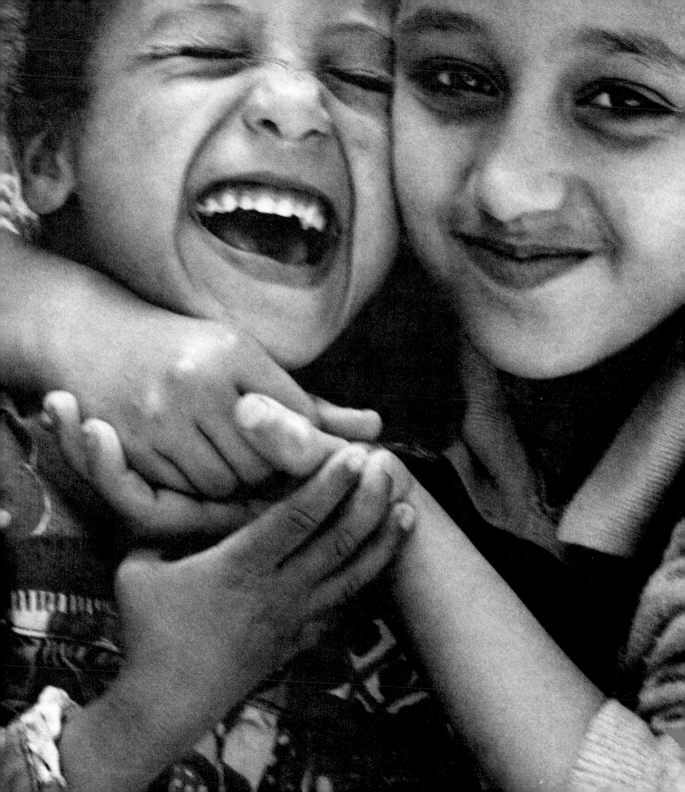

Moksha

Moksha is beyond *samadhi*.

It is the ultimate state of living in absolute freedom.

> In permanent awareness
>
> In permanent openness
>
> It is pure love
>
> True liberation
>
> It is divine.
>
> Forever.

It is the state in which the perceiver is simply a vessel, pure and uncluttered, for the channeling of divine energy.

Jesus and the Buddha are both examples of individuals who attained the state of *moksha*.

"... the Is doesn't even know about our illusions and games. It only knows Itself, and us in its likeness, perfect and finished."

RICHARD BACH

Illusions

I am the taste of pure water and the light of sun and moon. I am Om, the sacred word, the sound in silence, and the courage of human beings. I am the sweet fragrance in the earth and the radiance in fire; I am the life in all living beings and the striving of those who train their souls.

The Bhagavad Gita (VII: 8–9)

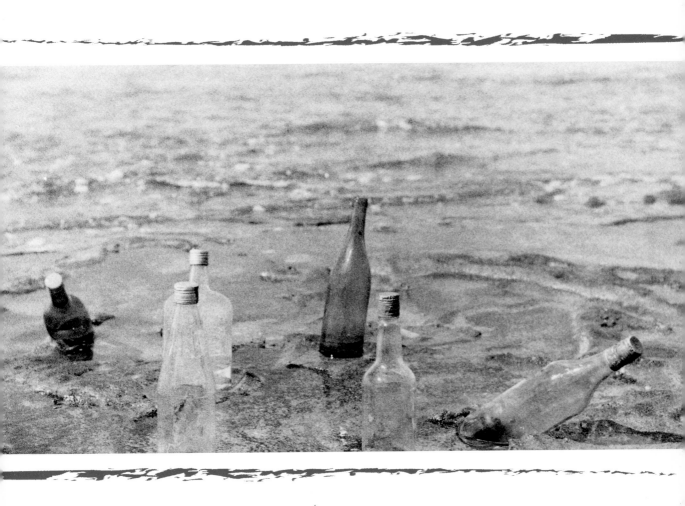

Adieu, dit le renard. Voici mon secret.

Il est très simple: on ne voit bien qu'avec le coeur.

L'essentiel est invisble pour les yeux.

ANTOINE DE SAINT-EXUPERY

Le Petit Prince

Bibliography

A. A. Milne, *Winnie-the-Pooh*. Methuen, 2000 (ed.)

Rumi, Coleman Barks and John Moyne (translators), *The Essential Rumi*. HarperSanFrancisco, 1995

Rainer Maria Rilke, Robert Bly (translator), *Selected Poems of Rainer Maria Rilke*. HarperCollins, 1981

Lao-Tzu, Stephen Mitchell (translator), *Tao-Te-Ching*. HarperPerennial, 1988

Eduardo Galeano, Cedric Belfrage (translator), *The Book of Embraces*. W. W. Norton, 1991

Peter Matthiessen, *The Snow Leopard*. Viking Penguin, 1978

Mary Oliver, *New and Selected Poems*. Beacon Press, 1992

Hillary Huttner (editor), *Mystical Delights*. Frontline Books, 1996

Czeslaw Milosz (editor), *A Book of Luminous Things: An International Anthology of Poetry*. Harcourt Brace, 1996

Federico García Lorca, Christopher Maurer (editor), *Selected Poems*. Penguin, 1997

Octavio Paz, Muriel Rukeyser (translator), *Selected Poems of Octavio Paz*. Indiana University Press, 1963

Karol Wojtyla, Jerzy Peterkiewicz (translator), Collected Poems: Karol Wojtyla.

Denise Levertov, *Poems 1960–1967*. New Directions, 1966

Rumi, Coleman Barks (translator), *The Illuminated Rumi*. Broadway Books, 1997

D. H. Lawrence, Vivian de Sola Pinto and F. Warren Roberts (editors), *Complete Poems*. Viking Penguin, 1994

Lucien Stryk and Takashi Ikemoto (translators), *The Penguin Book of Zen Poetry*. Penguin, 1981

Stephen Mitchell (editor), *The Enlightened Heart: An Anthology of Sacred Poetry*. HarperCollins, 1989

J. Krishnamurti, *Freedom from the Known*. HarperSanFrancisco, 1969

Rick Fields, *Fuck You Cancer & Other Poems*. Crooked Cloud Projects, 1997

Herman Hesse, *Siddhartha*. New Directions, 1951

Shel Silverstein, *Where the Sidewalk Ends: The Poems and Drawings of Shel Silverstein*. HarperCollins, 1974

Thich Nhat Hanh, *Peace Is Every Step*. Rider Books, 1991

Robert Hass and Stephen Mitchell (editors), *Into the Garden: A Wedding Anthology*. HarperCollins, 1993

e. e. cummings, George Firmage (editor), *e.e. cummings: Complete Poems 1904–1962*. Liveright Books, 1994

Special thanks to Bob Carlos Clarke for permission to include three of his photographs.